DATE DUE

BRODART

Cat. No. 23-221

THE DEVELOPMENT OF
AMERICAN PHARMACOLOGY

The Development of American Pharmacology

John J. Abel and the Shaping of a Discipline

JOHN PARASCANDOLA

The Johns Hopkins University Press
Baltimore and London

The Johns Hopkins University Press
701 West 40th Street
Baltimore, Maryland 21211-2190
The Johns Hopkins Press Ltd., London

Library of Congress Cataloging-in-Publication Data

Parascandola, John, 1941–
    The development of American pharmacology : John J. Abel and the
shaping of a discipline / John Parascandola.
        p.   cm.
    Includes bibliographical references and index.
    ISBN 0-8018-4416-9
    1. Abel, John Jacob, 1857–1938.   2. Pharmacologists—United
States—Biography.   3. Pharmacology—United States—History.
I. Title.
    [DNLM: 1. Abel, John Jacob, 1857–1938.   2. Pharmacology—
biography.   3. Pharmacology—history—United States.   WZ 100
A139p]
RM62A24P37   1992
615′.1′092—dc20
DNLM/DLC
for Library of Congress   92-11545

To my parents,

Ann and Louis Parascandola

CONTENTS

PREFACE

I first became interested in the subject of this book when I accepted a faculty position in the School of Pharmacy at the University of Wisconsin–Madison in 1969 and turned my research attention to the history of pharmacology. The emergence of pharmacology as a distinct discipline in this country, and the crucial role played by John Jacob Abel in this process, was clearly a story that needed telling. The existence of a rich cache of Abel papers at the Johns Hopkins University made the prospect of such a study even more attractive. I became aware, however, that a former student of Abel, Eugene M. K. Geiling, had been working for some time on a biography of Abel, and so I turned my attention for the moment to other aspects of the history pharmacology.

Professor Geiling died in 1971, however, without having produced his planned book on Abel, perhaps because, as K. K. Chen suggested, he was too much of a perfectionist (K. K. Chen, ed., *The American Society for Pharmacology and Experimental Therapeutics, Incorporated: The First Sixty Years, 1908–1969* [Bethesda, Md.: American Society for Pharmacology and Experimental Therapeutics, 1969], p. 1). Geiling did, however, collect much useful information on Abel and his family which was added to the Abel Papers at Johns Hopkins.

Although I had meanwhile become involved in studies on the history of chemical pharmacology, I began compiling materials on the history of American pharmacology as part of the Survey of Sources in the History of Biochemistry and Molecular Biology project in the mid-1970s. Much of that information was published in *Sources in the History of American Pharmacology* by John Parascandola and Elizabeth Keeney (Madison, Wis.: American Institute of the History of Pharmacy, 1983), and this work laid the bibliographic groundwork for my study of the development of American pharmacology. I am grateful to Merck, Sharp and Dohme Research Laboratories for providing a grant through the American Academy of Arts and Sciences to support the publication of *Sources*.

My research for the present book began in earnest in 1979 when I received a grant from the National Library of Medicine (LM03300), and additional funds from the Graduate School of the University of Wisconsin–Madison, to support the project. I spent the 1979–80 academic year as a Visiting Associate Professor at the Johns Hopkins Institute of the History of Medicine, where I had free access to the Abel Papers. I am especially grateful to the late Dr. Lloyd Stevenson, then Director of the Institute, for his support and encouragement of my work. Doris Thibodeau, then the Librarian at the Institute, and Nancy McCall, Archivist of the Alan Mason Chesney Medical Archives at Johns Hopkins, were particularly helpful to me in connection with my research in the Abel Papers. I have benefited greatly from the facilities and resources of the National Library of Medicine since joining its staff in 1983.

The research for this book was conducted in numerous libraries and archives, and it is not feasible to list individually all of the staff members who provided assistance. I would like to acknowledge, however, my indebtedness to the staffs of the following institutions: American Institute of the History of Pharmacy; American Medical Association (Special Collections, Division of Library and Information Management); American Philosophical Society (Library); American Society for Pharmacology and Experimental Therapeutics; Cleveland Health Sciences Library (Historical Division); College of Physicians of Philadelphia (Historical Collections of the Library); Francis A. Countway Library of Medicine (Rare Books Department); Food and Drug Administration (History Office); Johns Hopkins University (Alan Mason Chesney Medical Archives; University Archives); Eli Lilly and Company (Archives); Merck and Company (Library and Archives); University of Michigan, Ann Arbor (Bentley Historical Library); National Archives; National Library of Medicine (especially the History of Medicine Division); University of North Carolina, Chapel Hill (Southern Historical Collections); University of Pennsylvania (University Archives); Rockefeller Archive Center; E. R. Squibb and Sons (Archives); State Historical Society of Wisconsin (Archives Division); University of Wisconsin, Madison (F. B. Power Pharmaceutical Library; Middleton Health Sciences Library; University Archives).

Several articles based on my research for this project were published earlier. These publications, parts of which have been incorporated into this book, are as follows: "John J. Abel and the Development of Pharmacology at the Johns Hopkins University," *Bull. Hist. Med.* 56 (1982):512–27; "Development of Pharmacology in American Schools of Pharmacy" (coauthored with John Swann), *Pharm. Hist.* 25

(1983):95–115; "The Beginnings of Pharmacology in the Federal Government," *Pharm. Hist.* 30 (1988):179–87; "The 'Preposterous Provision': The American Society for Pharmacology and Experimental Therapeutics' Ban on Industrial Pharmacologists, 1908–1941," in Jonathan Liebenau, Gregory J. Higby, and Elaine C. Stroud, eds., *Pill Peddlers: Essays on the History of the American Pharmaceutical Industry* (Madison, Wis.: American Institute of the History of Pharmacy, 1990), pp. 29–47.

Many colleagues contributed to this study in some way, for example, by calling my attention to a useful reference or by giving me the benefit of their advice in discussions of my research. Again, I cannot thank them all individually here. I would like to acknowledge, however, those whose contributions were especially significant.

Elizabeth Keeney and John Swann compiled a great deal of relevant information for this study when they worked as research assistants under my guidance. Frances Kelsey provided me with an important collection of letters of Mary Abel and others which Dr. Kelsey had inherited from Eugene Geiling, and these letters have now been incorporated into the Abel Papers at Johns Hopkins. Henry Swain, of the Department of Pharmacology at the University of Michigan Medical School, shared documents and photographs concerning Abel that are in the possession of the department.

David Cowen read the entire manuscript of this book and offered insightful criticisms which I gratefully took into account in revising the work. My acquisitions editor at the Johns Hopkins University Press, Jacqueline Wehmueller, also gave the manuscript a critical reading, and her editorial suggestions contributed significantly to improving the book. Heather Boyd very capably copyedited the manuscript. I wish to express my appreciation to the following individuals for reading and commenting on parts of the manuscript: Thomas Bonner, James Cassedy, Harry Marks, and John Swann. The faults that remain are my own responsibility.

INTRODUCTION

The science of pharmacology involves the study of the interaction of chemicals with living matter.[1] It is thus a biological science akin to physiology, but it also has obvious ties to medicine and public health. Its practical applications derive from the knowledge that it provides about the therapeutic and toxic actions of substances.

Although the word *pharmacology* goes back to at least the seventeenth century in the English language, the modern science of experimental pharmacology did not emerge as a distinct discipline until the nineteenth century. Originally the word *pharmacology* was used in a general sense to refer to the study of drugs in all their aspects, including their origin, composition, physical and chemical properties, physiological effects, therapeutic uses, preparation, and administration. Sometimes the term *materia medica* was used synonymously with pharmacology, although *materia medica* was also often defined as the subfield of pharmacology that dealt with the natural history of medicines. The other two subdivisions of pharmacology in this classification scheme were *pharmacy* (the preparation and storage of medicines) and *therapeutics* (the use of medicine in treating illness).

In the nineteenth century, that portion of the science of drugs that concerned itself with the investigation of their physiological effects was sometimes labeled *pharmacodynamics*. During the course of the century, *pharmacology* was used increasingly to refer to this narrower subdivision of pharmacodynamics. The practitioners of this science came to call themselves pharmacologists.[2]

The broader meaning of the term *pharmacology*, to denote the study of drugs in general, has by no means disappeared from the language, and this has led to some confusion about what pharmacology is.[3] The subject is also commonly confused with pharmacy, the field and profession that deals with the manufacturing and dispensing of drugs. My focus in this book is pharmacology in the narrower sense, that is, the experimental science that deals with the study of the physiological effects of drugs or, more broadly speaking, the action of chemicals on biological systems.

By and large pharmacology does not have a distinctive methodology of its own. It may be differentiated from other biomedical sciences by its focus on the physiological action of drugs and other chemicals. One prominent pharmacologist noted that "the distinctive feature of pharmacology is not that it has any method peculiar to itself, but that it is ready to use any or all methods to elucidate the mode of action of chemical substances on living systems."[4] Or, as others expressed it in a recent textbook, pharmacodynamics (or pharmacology) is a "border science" that "borrows freely from both the subject matter and the experimental techniques of physiology, biochemistry, cellular and molecular biology, microbiology, immunology, genetics, and pathology. It is unique mainly in that attention is focused on the characteristics of drugs."[5]

Like physiology, pharmacology is heavily dependent upon experimentation with living animals. Classical pharmacology has emphasized whole animal research and, to a lesser extent, studies on isolated organs. In more recent times, studies at the cellular and molecular level have become an important part of pharmacological research. At the other end of the spectrum, pharmacologists have always been interested in the effects of drugs and poisons on man, and the ultimate goal of most animal research has been the application of the findings to human physiology. Only within the past few decades, however, has clinical pharmacology emerged as an identifiable subdiscipline of pharmacology. Similarly, pharmacologists have always been interested in poisons, but in recent decades toxicology has become a distinct subdiscipline, and some might argue that it is a separate discipline entirely. The development of clinical pharmacology and toxicology as fields distinct from pharmacology per se, however, occurred after the period on which this study is focused.

Pharmacologists have played a significant part in the development of certain techniques, such as those used in the physiological assay of drugs, but these are not necessarily unique to the discipline.[6] Pharmacology's theoretical structure is based upon physiological and biochemical foundations. If there is a distinctive pharmacological theory, it is probably the drug receptor theory, originally developed at the turn of the twentieth century by Paul Ehrlich in Germany and John Newport Langley in England. Neither of these men, however, considered himself to be a pharmacologist. Ehrlich defined his new chemotherapy as a part of the field of experimental therapeutics, and he criticized traditional pharmacology for focusing too much attention upon the study of the effects of substances on healthy animals. Langley was a physiologist. The receptor theory was not firmly established in pharmacology until it was developed in a more quantitative and useful form by pharmacologist A. J. Clark in the 1930s.[7]

Pharmacological methods and theories do not receive significant attention in this book. Rather, I look at the institutional development of the field in the United States. I am concerned with the transfer of the new science from Europe to this country, with how it came to replace materia medica in schools of medicine, and with how it became established in nonacademic settings such as industrial and governmental laboratories. Although I discuss many individuals and institutions, much of the book is centered on the role of John Jacob Abel as discipline builder. The extensive Abel Papers at the Johns Hopkins University are by far the largest single archival source for this study.

My approach runs the risk of overemphasizing the significance of one individual, but I believe that it is justified in this case because Abel was so central to the establishment of a discipline in a given country. Holder of the first chair of pharmacology in the United States, founder of the first American society and journal in the field, mentor of many of the early American leaders in the science, he is clearly the person most closely identified with the beginnings of pharmacology in this country. Abel has been revered by both his contemporaries and by later generations of pharmacologists as the "Father of American Pharmacology."[8]

The book is not a biography of Abel; it glosses over many aspects of his life and work. However, it does describe his education and career in some detail. The span of Abel's life (1857–1938) also tends to set the chronological boundaries of the story of this book. With a few exceptions, events covered by my narrative do not extend beyond Abel's death in 1938. The emphasis is on the period from 1890, when Abel was just completing his European training and about to embark upon his academic career, to the time of the First World War. This span of time was crucial for the establishment of pharmacology as a discipline in the United States.

In recent years, the emergence and development of scientific disciplines is a subject that has received significant attention from historians.[9] In the biomedical field, for example, there are the excellent accounts of the development of biochemistry (with some emphasis on the United States) by Robert Kohler and of American physiology by Bruce Fye.[10] This book is intended to serve as another chapter in the history of the development of biomedical sciences in America.

Although my theme is the development of pharmacology in the United States, I must at least briefly examine the origins of the discipline in Europe. Chapter 1 therefore begins with a consideration of the beginnings of a science of experimental pharmacology in the nineteenth century and how this new science replaced traditional materia medica courses in the Germanic universities. The chapter goes on to discuss the teaching of materia medica in American medical schools, and the early and unsuccessful effort to establish pharmacology at Johns Hopkins University.

Chapter 2 introduces the main figure in the book, John Jacob Abel, and considers his education as a biomedical scientist. Like so many other intellectually ambitious physicians and medical scientists of his day, Abel studied in universities in Germany, Switzerland, and Austria. He received his M.D. degree at Strassburg, where he worked in the laboratory of Oswald Schmiedeberg, one of the founders of modern pharmacology. Abel thus served as an important link in the transmission of experimental pharmacology from Europe to America.

In 1891 Abel returned from Europe to accept a position at the University of Michigan that can be considered as the first chair of experimental pharmacology in the United States. The third chapter deals with Abel's career at Michigan and at Johns Hopkins University, where he became the first professor of pharmacology at the newly opened Johns Hopkins School of Medicine in 1893. He held that position until his retirement in 1932. Abel's laboratory at Johns Hopkins became a major center for the training of the next generation of American pharmacologists.

Chapter 4 examines the spread of pharmacology to other American medical schools, with emphasis on the period through World War I. Case studies provide more detail on the transition from materia medica to pharmacology at three institutions. Some attention is also given to the development of pharmacology in other health science schools, using pharmacy as an example, and to the beginnings of graduate education in the field.

The fifth chapter considers the growth of pharmacology outside of the academic setting. The entry of the science into government and industry laboratories is discussed, with special attention given to the struggle of industrial pharmacologists to earn the recognition of their academic colleagues.

The final chapter describes the establishment of a national society of pharmacologists and a specialized journal in the field, with John Abel playing the pivotal role in both. A brief epilogue summarizes the consolidation and "professionalization" of the discipline of pharmacology in the United States and comments upon its present status.

The members of the professional society founded by John Jacob Abel must have been surprised to learn that the great man himself was to be the after-dinner speaker at their 1986 meeting in St. Louis, almost half a century after his death. The medium involved in this miracle was not a supernaturalist, but the medium of film. Those attending the meeting were treated to excerpts from a 1930 film of Abel delivering a lecture at Johns Hopkins. The film had recently been restored by Eli Lilly and Company and presented to the American Society for Pharmacology and Experimental Therapeutics. The appeal to members to participate in the event can serve as the invitation to this book: "Bring your colleagues and students for an excursion into the past and experience the historic relevance of a great pharmacologist."[11]

THE DEVELOPMENT OF
AMERICAN PHARMACOLOGY

CHAPTER ONE

From Materia Medica
to Pharmacology

The Birth of Experimental Pharmacology

Pharmacology as a discipline may be said to have had its intellectual roots in physiology and its institutional roots in materia medica. The science of experimental pharmacology emerged in many ways as an offshoot of the development of modern physiology, but it established its niche in the universities by replacing existing chairs in materia medica.

Although physiological experiments on animals have been carried out since antiquity, the birth of the science of experimental physiology dates back only to about 1800. John Lesch has provided an excellent account of the emergence of experimental physiology in France in the first half of the nineteenth century, focusing on the work of three key figures, Xavier Bichat, François Magendie, and Claude Bernard. Magendie has been considered by historians to be the principal founder of experimental physiology. It is significant that Lesch's book also discusses the beginnings of experimental pharmacology, and that Magendie's research on drugs and poisons is generally recognized as marking the birth of that discipline.[1]

The science of experimental pharmacology concerns itself with the study of the physiological effects of drugs and poisons, and it is therefore not surprising that its development is closely linked to that of physiology. As in the case of physiology, pharmacological experiments on animals had been carried out sporadically since ancient times. With the impetus given to biological experimentation, and particularly vivisection, by the work of William Harvey and others in the seventeenth century, a number of investigators undertook more systematic studies of the actions of drugs and poisons on animals. Among the more extensive and reliable series of pharmacological researches were studies on the action of various poisons by the Swiss physician John Jacob

Wepfer (1620–95) and the Italian abbot Felice Fontana (1730–1805).[2] Poisons were popular subjects of pharmacological research, presumably because the outcome was easy to measure, but one historian has commented that few of the studies of this period "contributed anything to pharmacology, the majority serving only to confirm that poisons were poisonous."[3]

As Lesch has pointed out, Magendie played a major role in establishing experimentalism as the basis of physiology.[4] Experiments on living animals were at the center of this research, and the vivisection techniques of physiology and pharmacology met with opposition from the time these fields began to emerge as systematic sciences. Magendie in particular became a target for such sentiments in the 1820s, especially in Britain, where the animal welfare and antivivisection movements originated. When Magendie presented public lecture-demonstrations during a trip to London in 1824, the *London Medical Gazette* reported that "a violent clamour was raised against the practice of experimenting upon living animals."[5]

Research on the physiological action of drugs and poisons formed an important part of Magendie's experimental program. His first experimental work, in fact, was a study of the action of upas tieuté, a vegetable poison from Java and Borneo, carried out in collaboration with Rafenau Delille in 1809. The substance was extracted from a plant of the genus *Strychnos* and was applied by the natives to the tip of their weapons for use while hunting or in warfare. Magendie and Delille also investigated the action of related members of the genus *Strychnos*, such as *s. nux-vomica*. For example, they allowed the extract of the poison to dry on a sharp sliver of wood, then inserted the sliver into the thigh of an animal and observed the effects.

The active ingredient of the *Strychnos* poison, the alkaloid strychnine, was not isolated until 1818 by the French pharmacists Joseph Pierre Pelletier and Joseph Caventou. Nevertheless, Magendie and Delille were able to establish that the spinal cord was the site of action of the poison, which produced convulsive contractions. When the brain was severed from the spinal cord, the poison continued to exert its action, but destruction of the spinal cord prevented the poison from acting. Magendie and his colleague were also able to provide evidence to support the theory that drugs and poisons are absorbed into the bloodstream and carried by the circulatory system to the site of action. At the time, it was widely believed that fast-acting drugs and poisons exerted their effects directly through the nervous system.

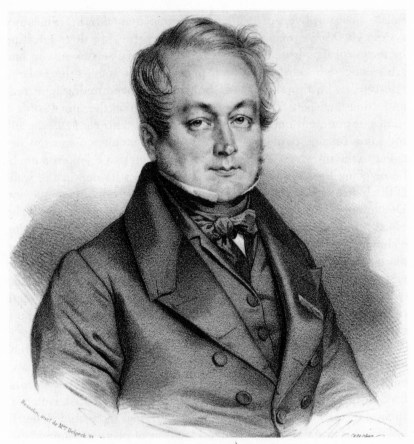

François Magendie, whose research helped to establish pharmacology as an experimental science.

Courtesy of the National Library of Medicine.

One of strongest arguments in favor of the theory of action through the nervous system was based on the belief that substances were not absorbed directly by the veins, but had to be absorbed by the lymphatic system before reaching the blood. The rapid action of some pharmacological agents was therefore difficult to explain unless it was assumed that their action was exerted via the nerves rather than through the bloodstream. An examination of some of Magendie and Delille's work on this point can serve as an example of the types of experimental techniques employed by the science of pharmacology.

In one set of experiments designed to test whether or not direct venous absorption could occur, Magendie and Delille attempted to isolate an absorptive surface from any connection with the circulatory system via the lymphatics. They isolated a portion of a dog's intestine by means of ligatures, severing all connecting vessels except for one artery and one vein. They then placed the poison in the isolated intestine, and within six minutes the symptoms of poisoning appeared, indicating that the poison had exerted its action on the spinal cord. A similar experiment performed with an isolated limb yielded basically the same results, demonstrating that this phenomenon was not peculiar to the intestine. To remove any suspicion that the poison might be reaching the circulation via small lymphatics hidden in the walls of the blood vessels connecting the limb and the body, Magendie and Delille cut these vessels and reconnected them by quill tubes. The blood transported by the artery and vein was thus the sole remaining communication between the limb and the body. Once again, poison placed in the paw of the isolated limb soon resulted in the usual symptoms. Magendie felt justified in concluding that drugs and poisons could be absorbed directly into the venous system, at least in some cases, although these experiments did not convince all of his opponents.

Magendie later carried out other useful pharmacological research, for example, investigating the action of tartar emetic, prussic acid, and emetine. His work on emetine, the active ingredient of ipecacuanha bark, was carried out in collaboration with the pharmacist Pelletier. In fact, it was his association with Magendie that motivated Pelletier to focus his interest in the chemical analysis of plant and animal materials specifically on physiologically active substances. In 1817, the same year in which Pelletier and Magendie reported their work on emetine, a French translation of Friedrich Sertürner's paper on the isolation of morphine, the first of the alkaloids to be discovered, was also published. Pelletier and fellow pharmacist Caventou developed a systematic research program for the isolation of alkaloids and obtained a number of important new alkaloids, most notably quinine, in the period 1817–21.

The isolation of chemically pure drugs played an important role in the early development of experimental pharmacology. Attempts to identify the site and mode of action of a substance were complicated when that substance might contain several physiologically active ingredients. Magendie saw a way out of the prevailing therapeutic skepticism of the time (which he shared) in a combination of the new chemistry with the new physiology. One could develop a more rational therapeutics through the experimental investigation of the physiological effects of chemically pure substances. Magendie even published a formulary based on these pure chemicals (primarily alkaloids) whose therapeutic value had been established experimentally. The first edition of the work contained only twelve substances, but it was well received and went through nine editions between 1821 and 1836.[6]

Magendie's pupil Claude Bernard helped to advance pharmacology as well as physiology. Bernard's brilliant studies on curare and carbon monoxide established the specific mode of action of these substances, helping to demonstrate the value of the new science of experimental pharmacology by providing an understanding of how drugs and poisons exert their effects on the body. In his work on curare in the 1850s, Bernard found that the paralysis caused by the poison is not the result of an action on the muscles—these may still be made to contract by direct stimulation—and that the sensory nerves were also unaffected. He further demonstrated that curare acted on the motor nerves, preventing them from stimulating the muscles (we now know that curare acts specifically at the neuromuscular junction).

Bernard's elucidation of the mechanism of action of carbon monoxide was the first explanation of pharmacological action at a biochemical level. He was able to show that carbon monoxide displaced oxygen in chemical combination with the hemoglobin in blood. This combination with carbon monoxide, which is extremely stable, prevents the hemoglobin from carrying out its normal function of carrying oxygen, and eventually the organism dies from oxygen deprivation.[7]

Magendie and Bernard helped to define the problems to be investigated by the new science of pharmacology, such as the site and mode of action of drugs. They also developed or refined a number of the experimental techniques of pharmacological research and demonstrated how these could be used effectively. However, neither Magendie nor Bernard expressed a desire to establish pharmacology as a distinct discipline. In fact, it is questionable whether they saw it as anything other than a branch of experimental physiology. Bernard, for example, seemed to be largely interested in poisons as tools of physiological analysis. By studying the mechanism by which the toxic agent caused death, one might hope to learn something about the physiological role of the tissues attacked.[8]

The establishment of pharmacology as an independent discipline, related to but distinct from physiology, required individuals who would devote their full time and efforts to the new science. These individuals were working in the German-speaking universities in the second half of the nineteenth century, and it was here that pharmacology began to emerge as a well-defined discipline.

The Institutionalization of Pharmacology

In medical schools, teaching about drugs had always been included to some extent in the curriculum as part of education in medical practice and therapeutics, but separate courses and chairs in materia medica evolved slowly. The complete history of the teaching of materia medica in European universities has yet to be written, and only an outline of its development is presented here.

The introduction of separate courses and chairs in materia medica or medical botany was tied to a revival of interest in botany in the sixteenth century.[9] Italian humanist scholars of the fifteenth century recovered and translated ancient Greek texts that had been unknown or relatively ignored in Europe during the Middle Ages. Humanists edited and translated the works of the four botanical authorities of antiquity: Theophrastus, Pliny, Galen, and Dioscorides. In the medieval Latin West, the botanical work of the last three had been known only through fragmentary, haphazard translations and encyclopedic compilations, while the *Historia plantarum* of Theophrastus had been completely unknown.

Renaissance doctors and naturalists recognized, however, that one had to observe living plants as well as study the texts of the ancients. For example, Dioscorides' *De materia medica* was the most influential of the botanical treatises of the ancients, but many plants of therapeutic value described by Dioscorides could no longer be identified, or there was disagreement over their identification. Humanist scholars made field trips to collect plants, started their own gardens, and traded specimens and seeds with other botanical collectors in an attempt to rediscover and add to the plants known to the ancients. As the sixteenth century progressed, plants brought back from voyages of exploration to the Americas and other parts of the world contributed to botanical knowledge. Scientific botany was further advanced by the publication of the first naturalistic illustrated herbals in the 1530s and 1540s in Germany, by Otto Brunfels and Leonhart Fuchs, as well as by the successive editions of Pietro Andrea Mattioli's commentary on Dioscorides in Italy beginning in 1544.

The renewed interest in botany in the sixteenth century, which Richard Palmer has claimed was "perhaps the most lively and fast-moving discipline" associated with the medicine of the period, found its way into the universities.[10] Given the importance of plant drugs in the materia medica of the period, it should not be surprising that the subject of botany first entered the universities in the medical faculty. The first chair of botany or materia medica (it is difficult to distinguish the two in this period) was created in the medical faculty at the University of Padua in 1533, followed by the establishment of a botanical garden there in 1545. In 1534, Luca Ghini was appointed as a lecturer in medical botany at the University of Bologna, and four years later he was made professor of the subject. Botanical chairs and gardens were soon established in a number of other European universities. For example, the University of Leiden's medical faculty attracted the noted botanist Rembert Dodoens to a newly created botany chair in 1583, and created a botanical garden.[11]

At first, the usual pattern of teaching consisted of lectures on Galen and Dioscorides (particularly the latter) and visual demonstrations of plants, supplemented by occasional field trips. Lecturers drew upon the botanical gardens of the universities where these existed, or sometimes upon their personal gardens or those of private citizens. Collections of dried plant specimens were also used in teaching, as were the shops of the apothecaries.[12] Traditions of medical chemistry and distillation originating in medieval times were given increased emphasis by Paracelsus (1493–1541) and his followers, so that by the seventeenth century chemically prepared remedies of various sorts also had a place in materia medica courses.[13]

The relatively small number of faculty at most European medical schools meant that the professors were often responsible for teaching several subjects, and they not uncommonly held more than one chair or a combined chair. For example, at Leiden, Hermann Boerhaave simultaneously held three chairs (medicine, botany, and chemistry) from 1718 to 1729. Although a stricter division of professorships according to subjects taught came about during the eighteenth century, so that faculty were not considered interchangeable with respect to their chairs, it was still common practice for professors to teach more than one subject. The teaching of materia medica and medical botany was frequently allied with the teaching of other subjects such as chemistry, as in Boerhaave's case.[14]

Although medical botany may have been an exciting subject in the sixteenth century, by the nineteenth century materia medica did not hold an especially prestigious place in medical education. A movement had already begun in the eighteenth century to reduce the number of remedies in the pharmacopeias by eliminating substances that were considered to be ineffective or associated with magic and superstition. The therapeutic skepticism popularized by the Paris and Vienna clinical schools of the early nineteenth century further called into question the value of many traditional drugs. Perhaps nowhere is this challenge to the value of the drug therapy of the time better expressed than in Oliver Wendell Holmes's often-quoted statement of 1860 that, with a few exceptions, such as opium, "if the whole materia medica, *as now used,* could be sunk to the bottom of the sea, it would be all the better for mankind, — and all the worse for the fishes."[15]

It is perhaps symptomatic of the relatively undistinguished place of materia medica in the medical curriculum that the man generally credited with establishing the first institute of pharmacology held a combined chair of materia medica, dietetics, and history and encyclopedia of medicine. Rudolph Buchheim accepted this chair in 1847 at the University of Dorpat (later Tartu), which was essentially German in its faculty and language although it was located in Russian-controlled Estonia. Born in Bautzen, Germany, in 1820, Buchheim received his medical degree in 1845 from the University of Leipzig, where he developed an interest in physiological chemistry. By the time he moved to Dorpat, he had extended his knowledge of pharmacy and chemistry through his editorship of the *Pharmazeutisches Zentralblatt* and his preparation of a German adaptation of Jonathan Pereira's classic English textbook, *The Elements of Materia Medica* (first published in 1839).

Buchheim argued that pharmacology, the science involving the study of the action of drugs, was a distinct discipline. "The investigation of drugs," he claimed in his *Beiträge zur Arzneimittellehre* (1849), "is a task for the pharmacologist and not for the chemist or pharmacist, who until now have been expected to do this." As for the more traditional aspects of materia medica, such as the description of the natural sources of drugs, Buchheim dismissed these as follows: "The pharmacologist has as little interest in the appearance of senna leaves as he has in the appearance of the case holding the scapels which he uses for his operations." He emphasized the need to isolate the active constituents of crude drugs and to determine their physiological effects on the healthy organism. Through such research, pharmacology would contribute to the advance of other medical sciences such as physiology, as well as help to establish a more rational therapeutics.

Shortly after his appointment at Dorpat, Buchheim established a laboratory and institute of experimental pharmacology, although at first the laboratory was located in his home and paid for out of his own pocket. It was only after about a decade that the university provided him with a laboratory in which he and his students and associates could work. Over one hundred scientific papers and dissertations dealing with the physiological action of various substances such as alkaloids and heavy metals emanated from his Dorpat laboratory. Although Buchheim's scientific contributions were not noteworthy, he played a significant role in the transition between materia medica and pharmacology. He articulated a concept of experimental pharmacology as a distinct discipline with a new class of practitioners and established the first institute of the new science.[16]

While Buchheim thus pointed the way toward a separate discipline of pharmacology, his influence beyond Dorpat was limited. He never succeeded, for example, in establishing a school of disciples to spread his ideas, although it was one of his students who played the pivotal role in the institutionalization of the science of pharmacology. Born in 1838 to a German family living in what is now Latvia, Oswald Schmiedeberg received his medical degree from Dorpat in 1866 for a thesis under Buchheim dealing with the determination of chloroform in the blood. Schmiedeberg remained at Dorpat as an assistant to Buchheim and was appointed the latter's successor when Buchheim accepted a chair of pharmacology at Giessen in 1869. At Giessen, Buchheim found himself once again without a pharmacological laboratory at the university, and he did not live to occupy the new institute that was eventually built for him.

Schmiedeberg remained only a few years at Dorpat, becoming professor of pharmacology at the University of Strassburg in 1872. The city of Strassburg, which had passed from German into French hands in 1681, had just been incorporated into the new German empire as a result of the Franco-Prussian War of 1870–71. A decision was made to reopen the German university, which had been closed after the French Revolution, and to make every effort to establish it as a leading institution of learning. An outstanding faculty was recruited, including in the medical school such distinguished names as Friedrich Goltz

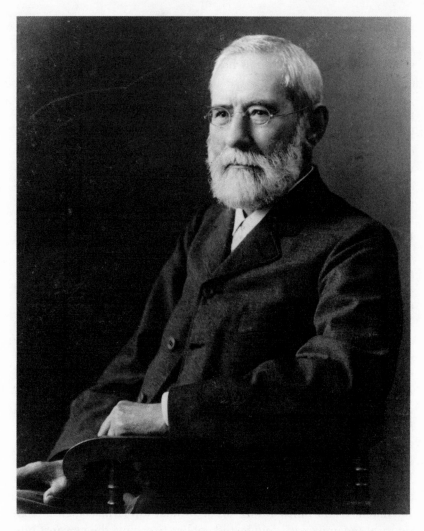

Oswald Schmiedeberg, shown here late in his life (1914), played a key role in the establishment of pharmacology as an independent discipline.
Courtesy of the National Library of Medicine.

(physiology), Felix Hoppe-Seyler (physiological chemistry), and Richard von Krafft-Ebing (psychiatry). On the recommendation of the noted physiologist Carl Ludwig of Leipzig, Schmiedeberg was appointed professor of pharmacology. Located in a major university with extensive resources, he was now in a position to significantly influence the advance of his field.

Schmiedeberg was provided with good laboratory facilities and later a large, well-equipped institute was built for him at Strassburg. While the research efforts of Schmiedeberg and his group, reported in more than two hundred publications, contributed significantly to pharmacological science, his greatest impact on the new science was exerted through his role as discipline builder. His institute became a mecca for students of pharmacology from around the world, the training ground for a whole generation of practitioners of the new discipline. More than one hundred fifty pharmacologists, many of whom went on to become leaders in the field, received their training in his laboratory. At the time of his death in 1921, some forty chairs of pharmacology were held by his students internationally. Among his more prominent disciples were Rudolf Gottlieb (professor of pharmacology at Heidelberg), Wolfgang Heubner (professor of pharmacology at Göttingen, Düsseldorf, Heidelberg, and Berlin), A. R. Cushny (professor of pharmacology at Michigan, London, and Edinburgh), and John J. Abel, the founder of American pharmacology.

In addition to his crucial role as a teacher of pharmacologists, Schmiedeberg contributed significantly to the institutionalization of the new science through the founding of the first journal devoted to modern experimental pharmacology (as well as pathology). Along with the internist Bernard Naunyn and the pathologist Edwin Klebs, Schmiedeberg established the *Archiv für experimentelle Pathologie und Pharmakologie* in 1873, shortly after his arrival in Strassburg. Schmiedeberg and Naunyn edited the journal until Schmiedeberg's death. Primarily pharmacological in content, it remained the premier journal in the field for many years and is still being published today as *Naunyn-Schmiedeberg's Archives of Pharmacology*.[17]

The first edition of Schmiedeberg's classic textbook of the new science, *Grundriss der Arzneimittellehre*, appeared in 1883, and over the next thirty years it went through seven editions and was translated into several languages. In the preface to the book, Schmiedeberg clearly describes the role of the pharmacological scientist as he saw it:

The following Text-book . . . contains in abstract only that part of the science of remedies upon which it falls to the Pharmacologist to form a judgement, and it is therefore neither a book of prescriptions nor a compendium of treatment. . . . The extent of and modern method of regarding Practical Medicine on the one hand, and Pharmacology on the other, do not permit the teaching of both subjects to be united in one person, on account of the danger that dilettanteism might interfere with one or other of them. Without pharmacological knowledge, the practitioner will always grope about in darkness as regards the application of remedies. To supply this knowledge is the task of the Pharmacologist. He is not, however, in a position to give directions to the Physician as to the treatment of disease; he must be contented, in formulating a science of remedies, to describe the actions of powerful agents in their practical application, more especially with respect to man, to characterise the consequences which follow the use of such means, under different conditions, for the entire organism, and from pharmacological facts to formulate general rules for the employment of remedies.[18]

Like Buchheim, and like later pharmacologists, Schmiedeberg insisted that pharmacology was a field distinct from therapeutics. He believed that experimental pharmacology should concern itself with all substances which through their chemical properties cause changes in the living animal organism, not just with those used for therapeutic purposes. On the other hand, pharmacological knowledge would help to form the basis for the development of a rational therapeutics.[19]

The conversion from materia medica to pharmacology began to take place at a number of other German universities in the 1870s and 1880s. One of the other German pioneers in the development of experimental pharmacology was Rudolf Böhm, who studied physiology with Fick at Würzburg and with Ludwig at Leipzig. In 1872 he succeeded Schmiedeberg at Dorpat when the latter moved to Strassburg. Böhm later served as professor of pharmacology in Marburg and then in Leipzig. John Abel attended his pharmacology lectures while a student at Leipzig in the mid-1880s.

When Böhm left Dorpat for Marburg in 1881, he was succeeded by Hans Horst Meyer, a pupil of both Ludwig and Schmiedeberg and another leader in German pharmacology. Meyer is probably best known for his work on the theory of narcosis. Like his master Schmiedeberg, he trained a significant number of students from various countries. In 1884 he again succeeded Böhm, this time at Marburg, and in 1904 he moved to Vienna. Rudolf Kobert, who served for many years as Schmiedeberg's assistant in Strassburg, succeeded Meyer at Dorpat, continuing a tradition of distinguished chair holders in pharmacology at the Estonian university.

A final example of prominent German practitioners of the new discipline of pharmacology in this period is Oscar Leibreich, who discovered the hypnotic properties of chloral hydrate. Liebreich became professor of pharmacology at Berlin in 1872, and a new institute for the subject was created for him there in 1883.[20]

By the time John Abel arrived in Germany to study medicine in 1884, experimental pharmacology had established itself as a distinct discipline, replacing materia medica at major German universities such as Strassburg, Berlin, Marburg, and Leipzig. The new science of experimental pharmacology had not yet, however, made a significant incursion into medical education in the United States.

Materia Medica in the United States

Materia medica was a part of American medical education from the beginning. The first American medical school, at the College of Philadelphia (later the University of Pennsylvania), included a series of lectures on the subject by John Morgan when it opened in 1765, and a chair of materia medica and botany was established there in 1768. And, as David Cowen has pointed out, "materia medica was an integral part of the curriculum of every American medical school established in the next one hundred years."[21]

Although materia medica was viewed as important enough to include in the curricula of all medical schools, it nonetheless ranked rather low in the pecking order of medical subjects. Cowen has noted that "only a few schools . . . were able to afford the luxury of a chair devoted soley to materia medica; more commonly it was taught along with another, often unrelated course."[22] Of course, in the early days of American medical education, when the size of the faculty was generally quite small at most medical schools, it was not uncommon for one professor to teach several subjects, just as was true in European schools. But even as the century progressed and medical teaching became more specialized, materia medica did not achieve an independent or distinguished place within the curriculum. The subject was frequently taught by faculty members whose interests lay elsewhere, and it continued to be thrown together with unrelated fields in a manner that suggested to Cowen that "these relationships were either matters of convenience or the result of a rather disparaging attitude toward the course."[23]

Although the teaching of materia medica could be combined with the teaching of botany, chemistry, hygiene, medical jurisprudence, and almost any other subject, as the nineteenth century progressed it was more and more commonly joined with instruction in therapeutics. The instructor in materia medica was also generally responsible for the teaching of pharmacy (i.e., the preparation and dispensing of drugs), whether as part of the materia medica course or in a separate course. Whatever the exact content of the materia medica course, it was almost invariably taught in a didactic fashion, the lectures closely following textbooks of the period, with little or no laboratory work (and certainly none involving animal experimentation until late in the century). Cowen concluded that in spite of European advances in pharmacology, in the United States "materia medica remained an empirical and traditional study, didactic in presentation, relying largely on botanical or alphabetical arrangements that depended upon memorization as the chief educational method."[24]

Late in his career, Torald Sollmann, one of the pioneers of experimental pharmacology in the United States, reflected on and summarized the status of American pharmacology (or materia medica) in the late nineteenth century, when he was a medical student.

> The subject was taught as "materia medica" through purely didactic lectures, generally by one of the minor members of the faculty who hoped it might be the stepping-stone to something better—a hope that was usually disappointed. And, naturally so, for what chance was there to show the mettle of a man by dry lectures on the botanical origin, constituents, traditional empirical uses, doses and incompatibilities. These mills ground slowly and very small and very dry.[25]

We may get an idea of the content of a typical materia medica course of the nineteenth century by examining a representative American textbook of the period, H. M. Bracken's *Outline of Materia Medica and Pharmacology: A Textbook for Students*, published toward the end of the century (1895). Bracken, professor of materia medica, therapeutics, and clinical medicine at the University of Minnesota, began by defining materia medica as traditionally consisting of the following subdivisions: pharmacognosy, pharmacodynamics (or pharmacology), toxicology, and pharmacy. In his introductory section, he devotes most of his attention to weights and measures, forms and means of administration of drugs, dosages, and prescription writing. There is a brief general discussion of the physiological action of drugs and some effort to classify drugs according to their action. These categories, however, are those of traditional therapeutics rather than those of modern experimental pharmacology. For example, the classes included alteratives ("agents which overcome certain morbid processes by modifying nutrition"), antiperiodics ("agents which lessen the severity, or prevent the return of certain periodic diseases"), antiphlogistics ("agents which tend to arrest inflammatory processes"), and tonics ("medicines which permanently increase the systemic tone by stimulating nutrition").

Following this introduction, the book is divided into six parts, where the articles of the materia medica are grouped not by pharmacological or therapeutic properties, but by their natural origin or chemical nature: acids, metals, nonmetallic elements, carbon compounds, animal kingdom, vegetable kingdom. A typical example of the description of a plant drug is that for belladonna. Bracken covers the parts of the plant used in medicine (leaves and root), the plant's natural habitat, its chief chemical constituents (atropine and belladonnine), and the taste and odor of the leaves and root. In discussing atropine, the most important active ingredient, he describes its appearance, taste, odor, physical and chemical properties, and dosage. He then briefly discusses the physiological action of atropine (its effects on the nervous system, on respiration, on the pupil of the eye, etc.), and concludes by enumerating its uses in medicine and its toxic properties (as well as the treatment for atropine poisoning).[26]

Although, in general, materia medica courses in American medical schools remained largely unchanged in character throughout the century, there were some American physician-scientists who were influenced by European advances in pharmacology and became seriously involved in pharmacological experimentation. For example, the prominent Philadelphia physician S. Weir Mitchell carried out a series of experimental studies on the toxicology of snake venoms and arrow poisons beginning in 1858, in collaboration with army surgeon William Hammond (who later became army surgeon general). After receiving his medical degree from Jefferson Medical College in 1850, Mitchell had traveled to Europe for additional medical studies, including a stint in the physiological laboratory of Claude Bernard. Although Mitchell never obtained an academic chair in physiology, he became, according to Bruce Fye, "one of the primary figures in the establishment of physiology as a discipline in America."[27]

Mitchell was no doubt aware of Bernard's work on the physiological action of the arrow poison curare, which the great French physiologist was investigating at the very time that Mitchell was in Paris. Curare was in fact one of the poisons studied by Mitchell and Hammond in their collaborative research. Using a variety of experimental animals, the American investigators administered curare by different routes and made detailed observations on the response of the pulse rate, respiratory rate, and temperature. Mitchell's extensive experiments on the physiology and pharmacology of snake venom, continued on his own after Hammond left Philadelphia, were published in a monograph by the Smithsonian Institution in 1860.

Although Mitchell can be said to have carried out pioneering work for an American in pharmacology, he can hardly be classed as a pharmacologist. As noted above, Mitchell failed to obtain an academic post in the fields of his first love, physiology, and had to make his living as a medical practitioner. His medical practice greatly limited the time available to him for experimental research, and his scientific work became increasingly focused on clinical neurology as his career progressed. That Mitchell, who was widely recognized as America's leading experimental physiologist in the 1860s, was unable to obtain an academic chair in the field is indicative of the difficulty of pursuing a career in medical research in the United States at the time.[28]

Mitchell's Philadelphia colleague and friend Horatio C Wood was probably the closest American approximation to a "professional" pharmacologist before John Abel returned from Europe to firmly establish the discipline on this continent. (According to Wood's son, his father's "middle name" was simply the letter "C," but most publications by or about Wood tend to place a period after the initial.) Born in Philadelphia in 1841 to a Quaker family, Wood received his medical degree from the University of Pennsylvania in 1862. He served as a physician for the Union army in the Civil War, and after the war returned to Philadelphia to work as a private teacher, or quizmaster, in medicine, therapeutics, and chemistry. Soon appointed to the chair of botany in the auxiliary faculty at Pennsylvania, he assumed increasing responsibilities at his alma mater over time. By 1877 he held the title of professor of materia medica and pharmacy, general therapeutics, and nervous diseases. The diversity of subjects in which Wood held chairs serves as a further reminder of the multiple responsibilities of many medical school teachers in nineteenth-century America.[29]

In addition to his teaching responsibilities and medical practice, Wood actively pursued research in a number of areas and published some three hundred scientific papers. He was one of the charter members of the American Physiological Society, and he was a strong advocate for animal experimentation in physiology, pharmacology, and therapeutics. His pharmacological studies dealt with the properties of such drugs as atropine, amyl nitrite, cannabis, ergot, ethyl bromide, and quinine. Particularly noteworthy was his investigation of the alkaloid hyoscine (scopolamine), whose pharmacological properties he was apparently the first to describe in the literature.[30]

Wood's famous textbook of therapeutics, first published in 1874, emphasized that therapeutics must be based on experimental pharmacology and physiology rather than on empirical knowledge alone.[31] The work went through thirteen editions and was widely adopted as a textbook of materia medica and therapeutics by American medical schools. Wood also served as editor of the *Dispensatory of the United States of America* for five editions beginning in 1883.

When pressure from the local antivivisection society caused the city council to stop allowing dogs from the pound to be used for research, Wood's zeal for experimentation led him to prowl the streets of Philadelphia in search of strays. He described his method in this way:

> At first I was nonplussed, but I soon designed a buggy, which could turn in its length, having a box in its rear; and owning a horse that had been trained for the racetrack, my colored coachman and I would drive through the purlieus of the city until we saw a homeless cur, which I seized by the back of the neck and locked up in the box, and in a moment we had whirled around the next corner and no one the wiser. After a time it became known that dogs would be bought at the University and we had no further trouble for a supply.[32]

Wood went on to indicate that he had a fondness for "well-bred" dogs and never used such animals in his experiments. He also emphasized that he always used "all proper methods to prevent pain and suffering." But he continued to battle the antivivisectionists, opposing them in many legislative battles in which he claimed he never "failed to check their mischievous designs."[33]

Although Wood was probably as close to being a pharmacologist as any American before John Abel, who received his baptism in the field in Wood's laboratory in the summer of 1884 (see chapter 2), he is best viewed as a transition figure between the old materia medica-

therapeutics tradition and the new discipline of experimental pharmacology. Like many of his predecessors, Wood held other chairs in
the medical school besides the one in materia medica. He practiced
medicine, in addition to his teaching duties, throughout most of his
career. His research interests spanned many subjects, and he was
probably as well known for his work in neurology as for his investigations of drugs and poisons. These diverse interests are reflected in
his bibliography of scientific papers, which has been broken down as
follows: 15 in botany; 14 in entomology; 54 in experimental pharmacology, physiology, and pathology; 12 in medical jurisprudence and
toxicology; 142 in clinical pathology, medicine, and therapeutics; 44
published lectures and addresses; and 10 popular magazine articles.[34]
Although Wood was a pioneer in promoting the value of experimental
research on the physiological action of drugs in the United States, he
cannot be considered America's first pharmacologist in the sense of
European models such as Schmiedeberg.

The Early Effort to Initiate Pharmacology at Johns Hopkins

The first conscious effort to create a chair in experimental pharmacology at an American university appears to have been at the newly
established Johns Hopkins University. The new university had opened
its doors in 1876, modeled on the German concept of a research
university. From the beginning, plans for the university called for the
establishment of a medical school. Although the medical school was
not scheduled to open until the Johns Hopkins Hospital was completed
(scheduled for 1887, but not realized until 1889), the university trustees created a medical faculty in 1883 to develop the plan for medical
education. The original medical faculty consisted of university president Daniel Coit Gilman, professor of chemistry Ira Remsen, professor
of biology H. Newell Martin, and John Shaw Billings, director of the
army surgeon general's library in Washington.

The Johns Hopkins University had already acquired a reputation
for excellence in graduate study and research. Not surprisingly, the
organizers of the medical school felt that it was "very desirable to
afford special opportunities for study and to encourage research in the
scientific branches of medicine." Among the scientific branches singled
out for study by the medical faculty at their first meeting in January
1884 was "the Physiological action of drugs."[35]

It seems clear that at the very outset the medical faculty favored the new science of pharmacology (the teaching of which had not yet been established at any American university) over the traditional materia medica. Physiologist Henry Newell Martin probably played an instrumental role in the medical faculty's decision to incorporate research and teaching in pharmacology into the program of the planned medical school. Martin was a protégé of the great English physiologist Michael Foster, and he had been recruited to Baltimore in 1876 as part of the original Johns Hopkins faculty. He was one of the key contributors to the maturation of physiology as a discipline in the United States. In an address delivered before the Medical and Chirurgical Faculty of Maryland in 1885, entitled "The Study of the Physiological Action of Drugs," Martin clearly presented the case for the importance of the new science of pharmacology.

> I have selected as my topic *Pharmacology*—that branch of science which is concerned with the investigation of the action of drugs on the healthy body—because I believe that it is destined in the near future to acquire an importance in regard to therapeutics which is not yet properly appreciated.
>
> Pharmacology can hardly be said to have existed in ancient medicine, nor indeed until the present century. . . .
>
> There are, at present, a small number of laboratories devoted entirely to such work on the continent of Europe; not one, I think, in the United States. Such investigations are, of course, often made here in physiological laboratories, but usually as a secondary matter and for purposes with no direct therapeutic end in view. I believe that as regards the advancement of medical art, there is nothing at present more desirable than an increase of well-equipped workshops, in which men already trained in chemistry, in physiology, in pathology, shall investigate the action of substances, with a view to discover whether they may be useful as medicines, and in what pathological conditions they may be rationally expected to prove of benefit.[36]

Except perhaps for his exclusive emphasis on the therapeutic goals of pharmacology, no pharmacologist would have found fault with Martin's description of their field.

Apparently a decision was made to try to secure an established scholar for the position in pharmacology at Johns Hopkins. Attention focused on two individuals, Thomas Lauder Brunton of London and Horatio C Wood of Philadelphia.[37] As stated above, Wood was closer to being a transitional figure between materia medica and pharmacology than a modern pharmacologist in the Schmiedeberg mold, and the same was true of Brunton. Both men, however, were clearly among the most prominent pharmacological investigators in the Anglo-American scientific community at the time. Brunton was lecturer in materia medica at St. Bartholomew's Hospital in London and the author of the widely used *Textbook of Pharmacology, Therapeutics and Materia Medica* (1885). He was also responsible for the discovery that amyl nitrite was useful in the relief of angina pectoris, and was one of the pioneers in the effort to relate pharmacological activity to chemical structure.[38]

Unable to obtain either Brunton or Wood for the position, the planners of the proposed medical school had to look elsewhere. While in Britain in the summer of 1884, John Shaw Billings discussed the question of the professorship in "experimental pharmacology" with several colleagues in London and Edinburgh, including Brunton and Thomas Fraser, professor of materia medica and therapeutics at the University of Edinburgh. They highly recommended Matthew Hay, who was then professor of medical jurisprudence and toxicology at the University of Aberdeen. Hay had received his medical degree at Edinburgh in 1878 with a thesis involving an experimental investigation of the physiological action of saline cathartics, and had served as an assistant to Fraser. Billings had an opportunity to interview Hay and "was much pleased with him." He informed President Gilman that, apart from Brunton and Wood (whom he was satisfied could not be secured), he believed there was "no better man for the place than Dr. Hay," and recommended his appointment.[39]

In October 1884, Billings wrote to Hay that he had been authorized to offer him the "chair of Pharmacology and Experimental Therapeutics (the precise title to be determined hereafter)." Hay was offered an annual salary of $4,000 with an understanding that he would not engage in private medical practice. He was ready to accept the offer, but raised the question as to whether he might not be allowed to devote an hour a day, or every other day, to private consulting practice, which he felt sure would not interfere with his university duties. The Executive Committee of the Board of Trustees denied Hay's request, however, stating that medical education in the United States suffered from the fact that the chairs were almost always filled by practitioners, with the result that the scientific work of the schools of medicine was "less efficient than it should be." They thought it best to initiate their own medical school by appointing several teachers who would not be engaged in medical practice.[40] Thus from the very beginning, the policy of full-time professorships in the preclinical sciences, then a novelty in the United States, was established at the Johns Hopkins University School of Medicine.[41]

As the Johns Hopkins Hospital was not scheduled to open until the autumn of 1887, and instruction in the medical school would not commence until that date, it was decided to delay Hay's appointment until 1 January 1887. In August 1886, however, Hay wrote to Gilman resigning his chair because of "private and personal matters."[42] No immediate effort was made to replace Hay, for it soon became apparent that the medical school would not be able to open on schedule. The university's income was severely reduced as a result of the financial difficulties of the Baltimore and Ohio Railroad, in which much of its endowment was invested, and the opening of the medical school was delayed until 1893 when funds were obtained from other sources.[43] Ironically, the person eventually hired to fill the chair of pharmacology, John J. Abel, spent the 1883–84 academic year (when the search that resulted in the selection of Hay commenced) at Johns Hopkins in the laboratory of Henry Newell Martin.

CHAPTER TWO

The Education
of a Medical Scientist

Boyhood and Undergraduate Education of John Abel

In the year that Oswald Schmiedeberg assumed the chair of pharmacology at the University of Strassburg, fifteen-year-old John Jacob Abel lost his mother to puerperal fever. Mary Becker Abel died in 1872, a few days after the birth of her eighth child, a girl who lived only to the age of four months. John was the first of the eight children born to George and Mary Becker, six of whom survived childhood.

In 1854 John's father, George, emigrated from Germany to the United States, where he went to work on the farm of another German immigrant, John Jacob Becker, near Cleveland, Ohio. George Abel soon fell in love with and married Becker's daughter Mary, and the couple moved to Cleveland, where George took a job in a rolling mill. Life at the mill did not suit George Abel, and he eventually returned to farming. He never remarried after the death of his wife, but raised his six children with the aid of a housekeeper and later with the help of his oldest daughter, Louise.

John Abel was born in Cleveland on 19 May 1857, and was apparently recognized as a talented student even in elementary school. He graduated as the top student in the Cleveland high school system.[1] Deciding to pursue higher education, Abel enrolled at the University of Michigan in the fall of 1876. Abel did not set out to study medicine, and the only science he studied in his first three years of college was physics, plus a little zoology and microscopic botany. At the end of his third year, his education was interrupted for financial reasons. Apparently, through the agency of a former classmate who had become superintendent of schools in La Porte, Indiana, Abel obtained a position as principal of La Porte High School in 1879. He also taught Latin, mathematics, and natural science in the school. After a year in this post, Abel succeeded his former classmate as superintendent of schools, although continuing to teach some science and mathematics. During his stay in La Porte, he met his future wife, Mary Hinman, who taught composition, history, and civil government at La Porte High School.[2]

It was also during the La Porte years that Abel made the decision to pursue a career in medicine. It is not clear what factors influenced Abel's decision, but his choice was made by the summer of 1881. Abel's teaching duties in science and mathematics at La Porte may have played a role in moving him toward a career in medical science. His interest in medicine was encouraged by E. S. Sherrill, a physician friend whom Abel visited in Detroit before proceeding to his family home in Cleveland for the summer months in 1881. Abel accompanied Sherrill on visits to several of his patients in their homes and in the hospital.[3]

In Cleveland Abel kept busy reading books on anatomy and physiology and performing dissections on frogs that he caught, as well as carrying out at least one vivisection experiment on a cat (using chloroform as an anesthetic). His father was not pleased with his choice of medicine as a career, believing the life of a physician to be arduous and precarious. Abel wrote to Mary, who was spending the summer with her family in Havana (later Montour Falls), New York, that ever since he was fourteen he had struggled against his father's "silent wish" that he make money—"mere money." He also hesitated to tell his father of his engagement to Mary, fearing that the senior Abel would not think him capable of taking on the responsibilities of marriage and carrying on his studies at the same time.[4]

From the beginning he was apparently more inclined toward medical research than practice, and recognized the need for a solid education if he were ever to achieve his goal of contributing significantly to his field. Late that July he wrote to Mary:

> It will be necessary to extend our apprenticeship over as many years as possible after leaving La Porte in order that part of the work that I have laid out this summer may be accomplished. I should be almost certain of finally seeing my great desire accomplished—that I might work out something—a masterpiece of some kind, in the medical line that will help people along a little—if I could have a few years of such unobstructed, uninterrupted quiet digging as I now enjoy. Of course, I would have to precede this period of digging with a training in laboratories such as I have not enjoyed.[5]

The remark about helping people is typical of the idealistic tone of many of the young John Abel's letters. He spoke to Mary of striving to live "the really high life, that so few can see the advantage of." He expressed a disdain for the "practical, pleasure loving, sightseeing" men who "become tradesmen of the most sordid kind merely." Abel was convinced, however, that he and Mary could rise above the ordinary existence, and that by sacrificing together they could "in the *end* do a little something for somebody, even if our actions should benefit only a dozen people." He asserted that brains were more important to his plans than money.[6] And he was convinced that intellectual excellence generally produced more good than did moral excellence. "A Harvey often does the world more good than a Luther."[7] In these letters one can sense a rebellion against his father's practical concerns for "mere money," another factor that may have impelled Abel toward an intellectual career.

By 1881 Abel had already begun to entertain the possibility of studying in Germany, which was widely viewed at the time as the international center of medical research. He also contemplated studying at the new American university based on the Germanic research model, Johns Hopkins. In the end, however, he decided that first he should complete his undergraduate degree at Michigan, and he returned to Ann Arbor in the fall of 1882. Much of his time during his last undergraduate year was devoted to studying physiology, anatomy, and physiological chemistry with Victor Vaughan and Henry Sewall in the medical school.[8]

Working with Vaughan and Sewall no doubt enhanced Abel's developing commitment to medical research. Victor Vaughan received one of the first two Ph.D. degrees offered by the University of Michigan in 1876 for work in chemistry. He then began teaching physiological chemistry at Michigan while pursuing the M.D. degree, which he obtained in 1878. Although Abel recognized the need to learn more chemistry and appreciated the opportunity to work with Vaughan, he was disappointed in Vaughan because Vaughan had little time to devote to his students. Abel complained to his fiancée Mary that Vaughan was so involved with private practice, editorial and consulting duties, and local political ambitions that much of his university work was delegated to his assistants.[9]

Sewall had more time for Abel and filled the role of mentor.[10] Henry Sewall received his Ph.D. from Johns Hopkins in 1879, working with Henry Newall Martin, professor of biology (see chapter 1). After completing his doctoral work with Martin, Sewall spent the next year in Europe working in the physiology laboratories of Michael Foster (with John Newport Langley) in Cambridge, Carl Ludwig in Leipzig, and Willy Kühne in Heidelberg. He returned to Johns Hopkins in 1880 to teach physiology, but was recruited to Michigan as professor of physiology in 1882. Thus he had recently arrived in Ann Arbor when Abel began studying under him. [11]

For part of the year, Abel spent all of his Saturdays in Sewall's laboratory, studying various animal tissues under the microscope with the assistance of the professor. Meanwhile, Sewall was also engaged in research with his assistant. In a letter to Mary, who spent the year at her family home in New York, Abel described one of these Saturdays:

> Today being Saturday was spent as usual with my microscope. My subjects were ganglion cells and nerve endings. Sewall and Hallowell were busy with their research work, experimenting on an anesthetized dog, whose occasional groans, however, it is comforting to think, do not result from pain. They usually have their dinners with them as they cannot afford to leave until the operation is finished. An outsider would be quite horrified to see them eating with one hand and with the other staunching perhaps some bleeding wound. One of Sewall's recent stories was about Prof. Burdon Sanderson, the famous London professor. He is a great tall, awkward man and one day while eating his dinner in his laboratory where he was experimenting with frogs, actually bit into one in place of the sandwich. [12]

From Sewall, Abel heard about the stimulating atmosphere at Johns Hopkins, which reinforced his decision to study there after completing his undergraduate degree. [13] No doubt he also discussed with Sewall the advantages of studying in European laboratories. Abel considered Sewall to be among the most fortunate of men because he had the opportunity to pursue a research career. Abel wrote to Mary in April of 1883: "Just think of being able to work out day after day one's theories as to the cause of this or that phenomenon." [14]

Postgraduate Work at Johns Hopkins and Pennsylvania

In June 1883, Abel graduated from Michigan with the degree of Bachelor of Philosophy. He married Mary Hinman that summer at his wife's family home in Havana, New York, and the Abels moved to Baltimore in the fall so that John could undertake graduate study at Johns Hopkins in the physiology laboratory of Henry Newall Martin. The Abels were delighted by the intellectual atmosphere and the laboratory facilities at the university but one can detect that for Mary, at least, Johns Hopkins did not live up to all of her high expectations. Mary had apparently hoped to study at Hopkins when the Abels first discussed going to Baltimore, and she was disappointed to learn that the university did not accept women.[15] Some months after their arrival in Baltimore, she wrote to a friend:

> This is the great American University and it must be advertised. Every man connected with it must have as many titles as possible after his name, must get into print by scientific reports, addresses, contributions to periodicals, etc. Tell me if you have seen the University Circulars or if they are in your library. If not I will send you ours. It's every word true, but somehow it is made to look larger than it really is. Now of course we ought to expect a great deal of incompleteness in an institution as young as this and it has really done wonders—but it seems to me the spirit is not what it should be. It is not the Faraday love for finding the truths of nature, the scientific enthusiasm which students even of ordinary mould may catch from a superior and work by all of their lives, it's a business like any other, with more or less emolument and honor connected with it.[16]

Although Abel's experience in Martin's laboratory was undoubtedly a valuable one, his desire to study in Germany continued to grow. Johns Hopkins University still did not have a medial school in 1883, so opportunities for study and research in biomedical science were limited. In addition, the lure of the German universities was strong for ambitious young Americans with an interest in clinical medicine or biomedical science in the last decades of the nineteenth century. Germany had emerged as the world leader in medicine, whereas American medical education was dominated by proprietary schools offering largely didactic lectures and possessing relatively low standards. Thomas Bonner, in *American Doctors and German Universities*, has discussed in detail why Americans traveled in great numbers to Germany to study medicine in the period from 1870 to the outbreak of the First World War.

So long as America lacked courses, laboratories, and instructors for teaching modern medicine, as well as public respect for both the science and practice of medicine, American medical men were forced to go to Europe and especially to Germany, the home of scientific medicine, for their advanced instruction. . . . What Americans found in the German universities was a revelation. In organization, spirit, facilities, and pro-ductivity the German university was reaching the zenith of its influence by 1870. Here were teachers . . . who were unequaled in their repu-tation for original investigation and patient teaching. The universities in which they taught boasted facilities which no American medical school could match in 1870. And there was an élan, a pride, a freedom in these universities which any American school might envy.[17]

Before going abroad, Abel decided to spend several weeks in the laboratory of Horatio Wood at the University of Pennsylvania in the summer of 1884. Abel referred to Wood in his letters to Mary as "the great therapeutist" and "the great drug man." Presumably Abel was drawn to Wood with the hope of learning more about therapeutics and pharmacology.[18] At the very time that Abel was working in his laboratory, Wood received an offer to move to Johns Hopkins as pro-fessor of pharmacology, which he declined. According to Abel, Wood was inclined to disparage that university and to praise the work going on at his own university, but Abel confided to his wife that, from what he had seen, Johns Hopkins was much more likely to become a part of "future science."[19]

Abel had only about a month of work with Wood on experiments involving the drug hyoscine, and no significant results emerged from his study. While Wood was impressed enough with Abel to ask him to stay in Philadelphia and become his assistant, perhaps attending medical school as well, Abel remained unconvinced that he should abandon his plan to study "pure physiology and all the essentials of medicine" in Germany.[20]

Leipzig and the Laboratory of Carl Ludwig

On 28 August 1884 the Abels sailed for Germany, with John in the possession of "a letter in exquisite handwriting from 'C. Ludwig' admitting him to that famous physiological laboratory."[21] Abel's plan for his German sojourn, and for his hopes for his future career, had been clearly outlined by Mary in a letter to a friend:

The plan now is to study abroad two years and then come back here for a Ph.D. . . . Two years ago Mr. Abel talked of medical practice as simply the profession nearest connected with the scientific study where all his interests lay. His aversion to putting his whole life into it has increased. Since we came here [Johns Hopkins] he has realized the backward condition of medical science as compared with other branches of science and the great advances that must shortly be made in it thus making necessary the better teaching of physiology and all that the medical practitioner applies. This would make it possible to continue investigation, to study more and more deeply. That Dr. Sewall had just such a place in Ann Arbor and the chance of working up a Physiological laboratory, that Dr. Vaughan united practice with his position in the medical college there, first made this seem possible. There will be more and more such positions in this country and men must be well trained to fill these. Certainly Mr. Abel's natural tendencies are in this line rather than in the "healing" art in itself.[22]

In 1884 medical education in the United States was on the eve of major reform, and preclinical sciences such as physiology, biochemistry, bacteriology, and pharmacology were to play a major role in revised medical curricula (see chapter 4).[23] Having studied at three of the four universities that Kenneth Ludmerer has identified as pivotal centers for the reform of medical education in the period 1871–93 (Harvard, Johns Hopkins, Michigan, and Pennsylvania), it is not surprising that Abel recognized that change was in the air and saw the likelihood of a growing number of positions for well-trained medical scientists in the mold of Sewall and Martin.[24] His work with these two physiologists inclined him toward the study of that science, and it is therefore also easy to understand why he chose the laboratory of Carl Ludwig as his German home.

Ludwig was one of the outstanding physiologists of his generation, and undoubtedly the most influential teacher in the field in the nineteenth century. His laboratory at Leipzig attracted students from around the world, including numerous Americans, among them such noted medical scientists as Henry P. Bowditch, Charles S. Minot, Franklin P. Mall, and William H. Welch, in addition to Abel.[25]

In a letter to a friend written shortly after their arrival in Leipzig, Mary reported that her husband was delighted with working conditions at the university and with Ludwig, whom she described as a man of "lovable character and wide intelligence." She went on to describe John Abel's workday as follows:

In the morning Mr. Abel works in the advanced lab. with nine others, under Prof. L. and his assistant—each has a different subject of work. Mr. Abel is on some point in nervous physiology. In the afternoon he hears lectures from Prof. Ludwig in Physiol. and Prof. Braune in Anatomy—twice a week also lectures from Dr. von Frey. The lab. is not as fine as the one in Baltimore—has not nearly the money in it, but is very perfect in every working detail. Both Prof. Ludwig and Dr. von Frey are there most of the time to advise and assist. (Prof. L's lectures are to med. students mostly—200 of them.) In B. Dr. Martin spent twenty minutes a day going hurriedly from desk to desk. Dr. Martin never did his own experiments. Professor Ludwig delivers the most thoughtful and suggestive lectures (tho' less perfect in style than Dr. Martin's read-off lectures) while performing the experiment that illustrates *every point*—tho' so old, long practice has given such an unerring touch that he almost never fails.[26]

Ludwig set Abel to work investigating whether or not there was a difference in the negative variation of motor and sensory nerves under heat stimuli. Although this work did not lead to any significant conclusions, Abel used it later in his dissertation for the M.D. degree at Strassburg. He soon became convinced, however, that he did not have the necessary background in biomedical science to carry out sophisticated research. Impressed with the broad and thorough background in medicine of his German teachers, Abel decided that he should largely postpone his research efforts and undertake more elementary studies in a variety of subjects, such as anatomy, chemistry, and even physiology. He therefore enrolled as a medical student, paying particular attention to the basic sciences and laboratory work.[27]

The Abels stayed in Leipzig for two years, and their first child, Frances Margaret (nicknamed Gretchen), was born there on 26 March 1885. In time, however, Abel became restless to sample the offerings of other German universities and he began to make plans to do so. The die was now cast for Abel to serve perhaps the longest German apprenticeship of any American of his generation, or, in the words of Robert Frank, to set the probable record "for gluttony at the intellectual table."[28] Entranced by the opportunities for study and research available to him, and possessing an unquenchable appetite for acquiring further knowledge and skills in preparation for a career in medical science, Abel found one reason after another to extend his European education. In June 1886, Mary Abel wrote to a friend (though she hesitated to inform her family) that they planned to extend their stay in Europe until the summer of 1889. By that time, she indicated, Abel would have received a degree (or degrees) as well as further specialized training, with the ultimate goal of obtaining an American professorship in physiology or pathology (united with practice, if necessary).[29] When the Abels had expended the money that they had saved for their sojourn abroad, John continued to finance his foreign studies through loans from his father against John's share of some family property.[30]

Abel's *Wanderjahre*

At first Abel was inclined to leave Leipzig for Berlin, but Strassburg was highly recommended to him and he decided to spend the 1886–87 academic year there. By this time, Abel had become convinced of the importance of studying more chemistry, particularly in its applications to medicine and physiology. Strassburg was home to Felix Hoppe-Seyler, one of the pioneers of the relatively new discipline of physiological chemistry, and Abel planned to work in his laboratory. According to Robert Kohler, Hoppe-Seyler's activities as a discipline builder were earning him and his institute an international reputation.

> Hoppe-Seyler was very active in promoting physiological chemistry. He formulated programs for the fledgling discipline, staking out a broad territory of basic chemistry, biology, and biomedical science. He founded and edited the *Zeitschrift für physiologische Chemie* (1877), which combined basic organic chemistry and a concern with biological processes. . . . For 30 years this was the only specialized journal of physiological chemistry. In 1877, Hoppe-Seyler published his popular and influential handbook, a major portion of which was devoted to basic biology.[31]

Abel was advised that he would be better off attending Hoppe-Seyler's lectures and working instead in the laboratory of the pharmacologist Oswald Schmiedeberg, who was also skilled in physiological chemistry but had a better-equipped laboratory and devoted more time to his students.[32] Thus Abel came under the influence of Schmiedeberg, who had played a key role in the emergence of pharmacology as a distinct discipline. On entering Schmiedeberg's laboratory, Abel was not totally without experience in pharmacology. As previously mentioned, Abel had his first exposure to pharmacological research in the summer of 1884 in the Philadelphia laboratory of Horatio Wood. While in Leipzig, he had attended the pharmacology lectures of Rudolf Böhm, another pioneer in experimental pharmacology.

Under Schmiedeberg's guidance, Abel carried out research in chemical pharmacology, for example, attempting to modify the toxicity of choline by manipulating its chemical structure. This work served to heighten Abel's interest in chemistry and his belief in its importance to medicine. In addition, Abel took the opportunity to attend the lectures of such noted Strassburg faculty members as Friedrich von Recklinghausen in pathology and Adolf Kussmaul in internal medicine.[33]

In spite of his preference for science over practice, Abel was concerned about the limited opportunities for pursuing a scientific career at an American medical school and feared that he might have to accept a clinical position. He therefore took advantage of the opportunity to arrange some work in German hospitals and clinics, spending the summer of 1887, for example, at the universities of Heidelberg and Wurzburg for this purpose. The fall of 1887 found the Abels back in Strassburg, where their second child, George, was born in April 1888. Abel also completed the requirements of the M.D. degree at Strassburg that July.[34]

At the same time, Abel began to think about his eventual return to the United States and where he might find suitable employment. In June 1888, he wrote to a number of his former teachers and other contacts to describe his training and interests and enlist their aid in locating a position for himself. He wrote letters to G. Stanley Hall, Henry Newall Martin, Henry Sewall, William Henry Welch, and Horatio Wood, among others, emphasizing that he would like to pursue an academic career in physiology, pathology, or pharmacology and therapeutics. To Sewall, for example, he wrote:

> As you know, I have been working for some time past at the *chemical methods* used in Physiology, Pharmacology and Pathology. I shall continue my education in this line. I feel tolerably at home in the Physical side of Physiology, and am trying to work up the chemical side. Of the theoretical medical branches Physiology of course is *my first choice*. My preparation is equally good for Pathology and Pharmacology and if a beginning in a good quarter offered itself in time I could devote the rest of my time in Europe to one of these branches.[35]

Abel was not yet satisfied with his training and hoped that he could accept a position with a delayed starting date, so that he could spend more time in Europe to specifically prepare himself for the work. Although Abel received encouragement from some of those to whom he wrote, no suitable position materialized at the time. Horatio Wood was actually somewhat cynical about the prospects for a scientific career, pointing out that science was "at a heavy discount in practical America" and that it was easier to earn $30,000 as a clinician than $5,000 as a physiologist. He noted that an academic career in medical science required great ability and talent and prolonged hard work. Even then financial success was not assured, whereas in practice there was an opportunity to earn a living on the basis of "respectable mediocrity or even intellectual poverty." If Abel persisted in his desire for work in science, Wood suggested that Johns Hopkins was perhaps the best place to go, in an apparent revision of his earlier critical view of that university. For clinical medicine, the larger cities offered the best opportunities.[36]

In October 1888, the Abels were dealt a grievous blow when their daughter, Gretchen, contracted poliomyelitis and died. This tragedy was particularly hard on Mary, who became greatly depressed. She confessed to a friend that for some months she even felt a repulsion toward baby George, begrudging him his hold on life, comparing his still "fumbling, half-unconscious existence" to that of his sister, so full of joy. She added that even though she had overcome that feeling, there was always a warning standing like a ghost between her and George: "Do not care for him so much—all is uncertain." The death of her daughter had brought home to her for the first time the uncertainty of the future, and the realization that from then on "there must always be tears behind the laughter and fear standing in the shadow of our hope."[37]

In the winter of 1888–89, the Abels left Strassburg for Vienna, probably glad to escape the site of their loss. One of the great European centers of clinical medicine at the time, Vienna attracted numerous American and other foreign medical practitioners and students to its wards and clinics. Still assuming that medical practice might have to account for at least part of his livelihood, Abel went to Vienna for further clinical training. Mary's sister Frances, better known as Franc, who was living with the Abels in Vienna at the time, described Abel's day, as well as his ambition, in a letter:

> Mr. Abel is working very hard and would be glad to do more if there were only more hours in the day. There are chances here in this great

hospital where there are always three or four thousand patients, to see and study every sort of disease that flesh is heir to—not excepting leprosy, of which there are two cases, brought from Bombay. He goes from one clinic to another all day and until nine at night when he comes home tired in body and sick at heart from all the dreadful sights he has seen. . . . I often feel sorry for Mr. Abel. He is so impatient to get at his work, feels so deeply the disadvantages of not having begun his preparation earlier, and yet sees just as clearly the absolute necessity of doing it thoroughly at whatever sacrifice. He has it in him to fill a first place in the profession, and it would be galling indeed to have to take a second or third for lack of a year or two of time now and the corresponding amount of money.[38]

Nothing tangible had come of Abel's letters to his colleagues in America, but he was content to remain in Europe and continue his work. The question of how to finance further studies continued to trouble the Abels, but this problem was temporarily resolved by an event that occurred in January 1889. Mary Abel had decided to participate in a competition for the best essay on the subject of "Practical Sanitary and Economic Cooking Adapted to Persons of Moderate and Small Means." The essay competition was supported by Henry Lomb of Bausch and Lomb, and was administered through the American Public Health Association. Mary submitted an essay dealing with the five "food principles" (water, proteins, fats, carbohydrates, and minerals) and included recipes and menus for providing a balanced diet at a minimum cost. The Lomb Prize Committee, which included Victor Vaughan and Ellen Richards, instructor in sanitary chemistry at the Massachusetts Institute of Technology and a pioneer in promoting science education for American women, unanimously voted to award the prize to Mrs. Abel over sixty-nine other entrants. The $500 cash award greatly improved the Abels' financial situation. The Lomb Prize was also soon to have other consequences for the Abels, as discussed below.[39]

Mary Abel and her sister Franc made plans to return to the United States in the summer of 1889, with John expected to join them in December. Franc was skeptical about this schedule, and commented in a letter that "this Abel family are so in the habit of staying longer than they had planned that I constantly suspect them." She thought that the "money question" would probably hold them to these plans, however. Mary and her sister did return to America as scheduled,

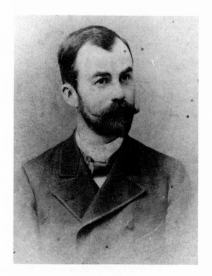 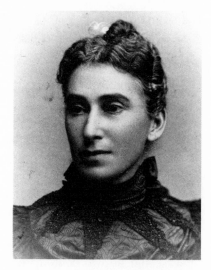

John Jacob Abel, Berne, Switzerland, 1889 (left), *and Mary Hinman Abel at about the same time.*

Courtesy of the Alan Mason Chesney Medical Archives of the Johns Hopkins Medical Institutions.

and John moved to Berne in the fall of 1889 to work with Marceli Nencki, the noted biochemist. He wrote to Mary that he was glad to get away from Vienna (presumably from clinical practice) and he hoped that his introduction "to American soil" would not be as a practitioner.[40] Even before he left for Berne, however, he was writing to Mary to plead that he needed to extend his stay in order to acquire the necessary level of expertise in chemistry, and asked her to see what she could do to borrow money from his father or their friends to enable him to remain in Switzerland.[41]

John Abel asked his wife not to think him "cold blooded" for wanting to stay abroad longer and he assured her that he felt their separation deeply. But he argued that "the all-important thing is more training," and expressed confidence that their "love and faithfulness" would prevent them from taking "the wrong steps just now." He envisioned a day when people could telephone cheaply across the Atlantic so that "lovers who are separated" as they were could "step up to the telephone every morning and evening" to talk to each other. Waiting four weeks for an answer to a transatlantic letter was frustrating to him.[42]

Abel was happy in Berne. He liked and respected Nencki, and

he thrived on the chemical research that occupied his days. Under Nencki's guidance he became more convinced than ever that chemistry was the key to the advance of biomedical science. He also recognized the crucial role that chemistry played in German industry. In the spring of 1890, Abel was writing to his wife and sister-in-law about a bold new project which he and Nencki were about to undertake, an attempt to synthesize "organized ferments" (i.e., enzymes) from "ordinary dead albumen" (i.e., protein). Abel viewed this as a first step toward the synthesis of life, though he requested his correspondents not to discuss this work with other members of the family or with friends lest they consider him a blasphemer. Although nothing of significance appears to have resulted from this effort, the incident reflects the exciting possibilities that Abel foresaw for the new field of biochemistry.[43]

In the meantime, Mary Abel also had an exciting opportunity. In October 1889, at the annual meeting of the American Public Health Association in Brooklyn, New York, she met Ellen Richards, who had been the first woman to attend the Massachusetts Institute of Technology, receiving a B.S. in chemistry in 1873. Richards was an instructor in sanitary chemistry at her alma mater at the time she met Mary Abel. Richards was also interested in the application of scientific principles to the study of home economics, and she had responded positively when the wealthy Pauline (Mrs. Quincy) Shaw, daughter of Louis Agassiz, offered to finance a study of the food and nutrition of working men and its possible relation to their use of intoxicating liquors. Ellen Richards decided to use this support, plus a grant from the Elizabeth Thompson Fund, to establish the New England Kitchen, patterned after the public kitchens in Europe. The purpose of the Kitchen was to experiment with the preparation of palatable foods that provided maximum nourishment at minimum cost, and to sell these foods to the working-class population of Boston for consumption at home.[44]

During a visit to Boston in November 1889, Mary Abel met with Ellen Richards and was offered $1,000 to go to Boston and operate the New England Kitchen for six months. The offer was almost certainly made largely on the basis of the Lomb Prize essay (for which Richards, as noted above, had been one of the judges). Mary accepted the position and the Kitchen opened for the sale of food on 24 January 1890. The idea was copied in other cities but was not a success, largely because the basically Anglo-American dishes prepared in the kitchens were not popular among workingmen of diverse ethnic backgrounds. The experience of running the New England Kitchen, however, proved to be a valuable one for the later work of both Richards and Abel. Ellen Richards became a consultant to various school systems, hospitals, and government agencies on matters of nutrition and diet. Both women played an important role in the founding of the American Home Economics Association and the *Journal of Home Economics*. Mary Abel served as the first editor of the *Journal*, which was founded in 1909.[45]

Mary Abel's income from the New England Kitchen project helped her husband to extend his stay abroad. Abel was anxious to prolong his European biochemical studies, and he suggested to his wife that if he remained in Switzerland she could join him and take courses related to her interests in food and nutrition. The Swiss universities of the day were unusually receptive to admitting women to medical studies, and Abel may have envisioned his wife taking at least some coursework in the medical school. Mary was willing to return to Europe, but wondered whether it might not be better for Abel to return home to make the personal contacts that would help him secure a suitable American position. She urged him to send copies of his published research to former teachers and other acquaintances who might assist him in his quest for an academic post.[46]

Mary Abel also took more active steps in attempting to further her husband's career. She attempted to make contacts on the Harvard faculty for him, and was most successful with Francis Henry Williams, who was a close friend of the Richards family. Williams, the son of the distinguished Harvard ophthalmologist Henry Willard Williams, was assistant professor of therapeutics at the time (see chapter 4).[47]

Williams agreed to see Mary Abel when she asked in May to meet with him concerning her husband's career. Having himself studied in Europe for two years, including a stint in Schmiedeberg's laboratory, Williams was favorably disposed toward Abel and told Mary he would be willing to take him on as an assistant in his laboratory research and clinical work. She indicated that her husband's current interests were running more toward physiological chemistry than pharmacology, but Williams was willing to be somewhat flexible about the scope of the research, and pointed out that the boundary between the two subjects was blurred, especially in the United States. Experimental therapeutics, he argued, was a broad field.[48]

At about that same time Mary received a letter from the Reighards, friends in Ann Arbor, informing her that Victor Vaughan was thinking of giving up his physiological chemistry teaching due to the press of his other duties. Jacob Reighard, assistant professor of zoology at Michigan, had mentioned to Vaughan that John Abel was planning to return to this country and was seeking a position. Mary immediately informed her husband of this possible opportunity, and also wrote to Vaughan herself asking him to write to Abel with any information concerning an opening at Michigan. Coincidentally, Abel wrote to Vaughan at about this same time, basically to seek his assistance in locating a position at an American medical school.[49]

In the end, Vaughan did offer Abel the opportunity to teach physiological chemistry at Michigan, but Abel declined for a variety of reasons. He had already written to Williams to accept the Harvard assistantship just before he learned of the possibility in Ann Arbor, but later circumstances would reveal that this in itself would not have deterred him from accepting Vaughan's offer. Other factors were of more significance in the decision. Vaughan was apparently vague about the salary, which Abel presumed to be small, and about the level and responsibilities of the position. There was also some discussion of histology (which Abel disliked) being made a component of his work. Finally, when Abel received Vaughan's letter in late June, he was preparing to leave Nencki's laboratory shortly for a tour of various European laboratories before returning to the United States in September, and he did not think there was time for him to resolve these concerns. Abel suggested that once he was back in this country he could arrange to discuss the matter further with Vaughan if the position were still open for the following year.[50]

Thus, in early June 1890, Abel's plans for the next year appeared to be settled. After visiting several more European laboratories, he would finally return home in September to take up a position as an assistant to Williams in Boston, expecting to do research in experimental pharmacology and therapeutics. He expressed the hope to Mary that he could "work up this newest and most fruitful branch of medical science to the position it deserves in every medical school where more than the technique of medical practice is taught."[51] As he was preparing to leave Berne, however, another letter arrived from Vaughan which caused Abel to alter these plans.[52] The letter, which arrived on July 15, read as follows: "How would the chair of materia medica and therapeutics suit you, say with physiological chemistry attached? This chair is now vacant. Just how much clinical work have you done? If this would suit you, send me all the references you can get immediately. The Board meets on the 28th of this month and desires to fill this place at that time."[53]

The University of Michigan had had a professor of materia medica since 1848, although the course was apparently not taught until after the medical school admitted its first students in 1850. From the beginning, the teaching of the subject was generally combined with other duties. For example, materia medica was included in the title of George E. Frothingham's position from 1876 until he resigned from the faculty in 1889, but at various times he also simultaneously held other professorships in subjects such as practical anatomy, ophthalmology, and aural surgery. For part of that period, he did not actually teach materia medica, despite holding the chair in that subject. A history of the university has noted that during the first forty years of the medical department, "the teaching of materia medica and therapeutics had been combined with some other discipline. Like a poor relative it was passed around from one professor to another. Thus, during four decades the names of ten men, from Douglas to Georg, were associated with materia medica and therapeutics."[54]

As we have seen, this was a typical pattern for the teaching of that subject in nineteenth-century American medical schools. Although Frothingham held the chair of materia medica (among other subjects) in 1889, the materia medica course was apparently taught by an instructor named Conrad Georg.[55]

Frothingham was essentially forced out because of his strenuous opposition to the construction of a new university hospital in Ann Arbor. He was part of a faction of the Michigan faculty that had been advocating the move of the medical school to Detroit, where they believed improved clinical facilities would be available. The building of a new hospital in Ann Arbor would have made a move to Detroit unlikely. Frothingham and professor of surgery Donald Maclean went so far in their opposition to the hospital that the university's Board of Regents invited them to turn in their resignations. Frothingham resigned in 1889, thereby vacating the chair of materia medica which was to be offered to Abel one year later.[56]

CHAPTER THREE

Abel and the Beginnings of
Pharmacology in American Medical Schools

Abel at Michigan

John Abel had not set out to be a pharmacologist. Indeed, the field hardly existed as an experimental science in the United States at the time he took up his studies in Germany. During his medical studies abroad, however, he became familiar with the new science as practiced in a university setting by respected scientists such as Schmiedeberg, and recognized that he could fashion a career for himself in pharmacology as well as in physiology or physiological chemistry. Therefore, Vaughan's offer of the chair of materia medica and therapeutics at Michigan in July 1890 was attractive to Abel, and after consulting with Nencki he cabled Vaughan with his acceptance. Less than a month after accepting the position, he was already cautioning Mary Abel that they would have to live economically because he planned on further study in the future, and he added: "I mean to do still better than A. A. [Ann Arbor] *between you and me.*"[1]

Abel's letters to his wife at the time suggest that he had come to the conclusion that pharmacology, presumably because of its practical applications in therapeutics, was a more promising field than physiological chemistry for career advancement in the United States (though of course there may have been a certain amount of rationalization in his reasoning). After receiving the Michigan offer, for example, he wrote to Mary: "Pharmacology is a better line [than physiological chemistry] in America at present."[2] in another letter to her he stated: "Chemistry is as necessary in Pharmacology or what we call Therapeutics as it is in Physiological Chemistry. And I know that I can make vastly more out of Pharmacology in the States."[3] Abel also recalled years later that Nencki had encouraged him to accept the position, even though he had not originally planned to become a pharmacologist, since the subject was one of the broadest fields of medicine and could be approached from many points of view.[4]

Abel followed up his cablegram to Vaughan with a letter indicating that there was one condition for his acceptance of the position, namely, that his appointment not take effect until at least 1 January 1891, so that he could extend his stay in Europe to study further the "practical, bedside" aspect of therapeutics. He expressed confidence that he could manage the theoretical and experimental part of his teaching responsibilities, since he had devoted significant time to the work underlying therapeutics ("what the Germans call pharmacology"), but he confessed that he did not have much experience in the art of prescribing medicines. To Mary, he admitted that he could back down on this condition if necessary, but that he preferred to go better prepared, once again typical of his desire to prolong his European apprenticeship. He also commented to her that there were no young men in the United States trained in pharmacology, and that if they were "fools enough" at Michigan to take an "old man" (i.e., a practitioner) they would simply fall behind other schools (presumably schools with vision enough to hire someone like Abel).[5] Although Abel's request was granted, he actually spent much of the fall of 1890 in the laboratory of the biochemist Edmund Drechsel at Leipzig, further enhancing his chemical skills— a reflection of his continued preference for the laboratory over the clinic.[6]

At Abel's request, Nencki, Ludwig, Schmiedeberg, and Bernard Naunyn (professor of internal medicine at Strassburg) sent letters of reference to Michigan on his behalf. His appointment was approved by the Board of Regents, with a starting date of 1 January 1891 and an annual salary of $2,000. He had no difficulty in extricating himself from his agreement to work for Williams at Harvard. Meanwhile Vaughan had decided not to add physiological chemistry, as originally intended, to Abel's responsibilities so as not to overburden him (since Abel had expressed some concern about the teaching load). There was also some confusion about the level of Abel's appointment, as he was expecting a professorship and was only appointed as a lecturer. He was assured, however, that such an arrangement was typical for the first year of appointment at Michigan, and that he would be promoted to professor in his second year if his performance was satisfactory.[7]

After completing his European studies, Abel arrived in Ann Arbor in early January 1891. Although the traditional title of "materia medica and therapeutics" was retained for his position, his appointment at Michigan must be considered the first professorship of experimental pharmacology in the United States. Abel's appointment, as we have seen, came about through a combination of fortuitous circumstances (including Frothingham's resignation and Abel's former ties with Michigan). Although Vaughan deserves the credit for hiring Abel, the version of the appointment given in Vaughan's autobiography, emphasizing his own foresightedness, is inaccurate. According to Vaughan:

When in 1890 we decided to have a real chair of pharmacology with laboratory instruction, I wrote to Professor Oswald Schmiedeberg, the dean of that science at that time in Strasbourg. He replied at length and advised me not to take a German, since he thought it a doubtful procedure to install a foreigner into a professorship. He said that he had in his laboratory two Americans but that one of them was more German than American and he recommended the other. Besides, he said that the man he was recommending was not only an American but a graduate of Michigan University. In this way John J. Abel became our first professor of pharmacology, as a real science.[8]

As we have seen, the chain of events leading to Abel's appointment did not occur just this way. It was the Abels who first contacted Vaughan about a possible position at Michigan, and Vaughan's initial offer to Abel involved only the teaching of physiological chemistry. At the time Abel was working in Nencki's laboratory in Berne, and not with Schmiedeberg, having in fact left Strassburg in the winter of 1888–89. Schmiedeberg apparently wrote to Vaughan at Abel's request. The evidence does not suggest that Vaughan had decided to convert the materia medica position to one in modern pharmacology before Abel contacted him in 1890. It is possible, of course, that Vaughan, who was most likely aware of the development of experimental pharmacology in German universities, had such a plan in mind, but he does not appear to have taken any definite steps in that direction before employing Abel.[9] It may be that Abel's training in physiological chemistry played more of a role in his being hired than any specific plan by Vaughan about the nature of the materia medica position. In informing Abel about his appointment by the Board of Regents, Vaughan claimed that Michigan would be especially strong in chemistry, which he saw as eventually eclipsing bacteriology in importance for medicine, and that he kept this fact in mind in selecting new faculty for the medical school.[10]

Abel brought to Michigan the German tradition of experimental pharmacology as molded by Buchheim and Schmiedeberg. As he phrased it years later: "Here at Ann Arbor I was given the opportunity of starting the first professorship of pharmacology in the United States, whose holder should devote himself entirely to giving students the best possible instruction by means of lectures, demonstrations and quizzes, in the manner in which my European teachers (Schmiedeberg and Boehm) had long carried on their work."[11] Conditions for teaching or research in experimental pharmacology at Michigan were not what Abel had experienced in Germany. He recalled that, when he arrived in Ann Arbor, there was no laboratory of any kind at his disposal:

> There was not a scrap of apparatus, not even a test-tube, a flask or a beaker. All these things, when I needed them, had to be borrowed, for the first weeks. . . . The only material evidence that the School had ever had a department of materia medica and therapeutics was to be found in a large collection of official drugs, contained in beautiful glass jars that had been bought in France many years before.[12]

Abel transformed the traditional materia medica course at Michigan into a course on pharmacology, which included vivisection demonstrations to illustrate his lectures. Some of these demonstrations had to be given in the surgical amphitheater rather than in the room where Abel usually lectured. After his first year of teaching, Abel also made arrangements for the pharmacy and dentistry students who had been in his course to receive instruction in pharmacology in their own schools because he believed they did not have the necessary background in physiology and medicine to take the course that he taught. At that same time, he arranged to have the course moved from the first to the third year of the medical curriculum, presumably so that students in his course would have already taken physiology and physiological chemistry, which were offered in the second year. A background in physiology had not been deemed necessary for a course in materia medica, but clearly Abel believed it was required preparation for instruction in pharmacology.

Abel also took immediate steps to establish a laboratory in which he could pursue his research interests. A small laboratory was set up under the stairs leading to the amphitheater where most of the medical lectures were given. A senior medical student from Canada, Archibald Muirhead (later professor of pharmacology, physiology, and materia medica at Creighton University College of Medicine) served as Abel's assistant. Besides assisting Abel in his research and in the experimental

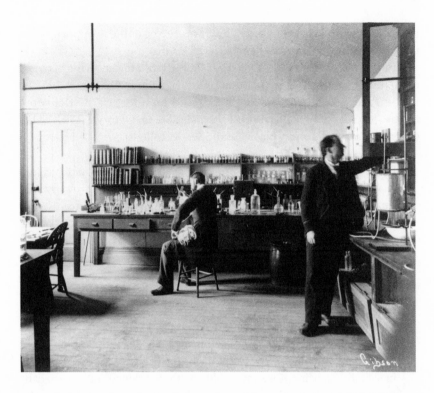

John Abel (seated in the background) *and his assistant, Archibald Muir-head, in Abel's pharmacology laboratory at the University of Michigan about 1891.*

Courtesy of the Bentley Historical Library, University of Michigan, Ann Arbor.

demonstrations used in teaching, Muirhead lived with the Abels and handled certain domestic chores, such as taking care of the furnace. As noted, Abel inherited essentially no laboratory equipment from his predecessor and had to borrow what he could at first. The university allotted him the relatively generous sum of $900, however, to purchase equipment and supplies during his first year in Ann Arbor, as well as soon providing him with the space for a larger laboratory.

During his second year at Michigan, Abel also introduced two advanced laboratory courses designed for graduate students, one on the influence of drugs on metabolism and the other on methods of modern pharmacology. In addition, he organized a journal club, which he invited about fifteen of the better students in the medical class to join, and announced his willingness to have advanced students undertake research projects in his laboratory. Unfortunately, there is no record of how many students availed themselves of these opportunities for advanced coursework or research.[13]

It was also at this time that Abel first articulated in print his view of the new science of experimental pharmacology in a paper published in the *Pharmaceutical Era* in 1892, based on a lecture he delivered to the Michigan Pharmaceutical Association in October 1891. Abel described pharmacology to his audience as follows:

> Briefly this science tries to discover all the chemical and physical changes that go on in a living thing that has absorbed a substance capable of producing such changes, and it also attempts to discover the fate of the substance incorporated. It is not therefore an applied science, like therapeutics, but it is one of the biological sciences, using that word in its widest sense. Like its sister sciences, physiology, physiological chemistry and pathology, it is making great progress along certain physical and chemical lines, which is pioneer work of a necessary kind toward an explanation of vital processes. . . .
>
> It was such experiments as these that led Buchheim and others to insist on the insufficiency of the mere bedside study of medicines, and led to the erection of special pharmacological laboratories . . . in which experimenters can build up their science undisturbed by the intrusive demands of practical utility. But pharmacology once on a firm basis will yield valuable results for the practical man.[14]

In this statement Abel was expressing a philosophy characteristic of the first generations of pharmacologists. Pharmacology was not an applied science, like therapeutics, but a basic biological science akin to physiology. The field could not advance as a science as long as it was tied to the bedside and was seen as a "handmaiden to therapeutics." On the other hand, Abel and his colleagues did not wish to imply that pharmacology would produce no practical benefits. If the discipline were allowed to grow and flourish in pharmacological laboratories and institutes, it would eventually yield results that would be applicable to the practice of medicine.

Abel's lecture was accompanied by several experimental demonstrations designed to illustrate some of the methods of pharmacological research. For example, one demonstration involved observation of the effects of various chemical agents upon the vascular mechanism of the rabbit. An anesthetized rabbit was paralyzed with curare to eliminate any disturbing influences of muscular movements. Because the curare prevented the respiratory muscles from functioning, Abel's assistant had to keep the animal breathing by means of a bellows connected directly to the trachea of the rabbit. A glass cannula was inserted into the carotid artery of the rabbit and the arterial blood rose to a height of four to five feet in the tube. The height of the blood in the tube served as a measurement of arterial blood pressure. When the animal was allowed to inhale a few drops of chloroform, the blood pressure dropped rapidly. Abel explained that this decrease in pressure was due to vasodilation of the peripheral arteries, caused by chloroform's paralyzing action on the vasomotor center in the brain, which normally exercises a tonic, constricting influence on the arteries. Ammonia, on the other hand, reverses the action of chloroform and causes the blood pressure to rise, as Abel demonstrated.[15]

During his brief tenure at Michigan, Abel embarked upon several research investigations, two of them particularly reflecting his interest in chemistry and his conviction of its importance to medicine. With Muirhead he began the work that later (after he moved to Johns Hopkins) led him to demonstrate that ethyl sulfide is a constituent of dog urine and was responsible for the strong unpleasant odor produced during ammonia determinations on dog urine. Also working with Muirhead, Abel explained the presence of free ammonia in the urine of children who had received large amounts of lime water, used to treat diarrhea. The lime water (a solution of calcium hydroxide) led to the presence of calcium carbamate in the urine, which Abel had earlier found in horse's urine in his work with Drechsel. The calcium carbamate readily decomposed to calcium carbonate, carbon dioxide, and ammonia.[16]

In the summer of 1892, unable to resist the lure of Europe, Abel returned to work with Drechsel again, this time at Berne where the latter had moved to replace Nencki, who had accepted a position in St. Petersburg, Russia. In a letter to Mary, who remained at home, Abel confessed that he no longer thought he could live in Europe, adding: "I dare say it is you and the boys and the fact that I have been fairly successful at Ann Arbor that are responsible for the different feeling."[17] While abroad he also took the opportunity to purchase European equipment for his Michigan laboratory.[18]

Although Abel wrote years later that soon after he arrived in Ann Arbor, "after a few medical consultations and the taking over of my old friend Herdmann's practice for ten days while he was away on a vacation, I decided that it was impossible to serve two masters, and so dropped all idea of carrying on work in internal medicine and devoted myself entirely to my subject [pharmacology]," it is evident that in the summer of 1892 he still had some ambivalence about completely abandoning clinical work.[19] When Michigan gave him leave to remain in Europe until November, he wrote to Mary that he ought to go to Vienna and "pick up medicine" and perhaps give up his plans to do pharmacological work in Basel and Strassburg. Once again, however, his scientific interests won out and he convinced himself that it was more important to concentrate on pharmacological methods for the book that he was planning to write (but never did). It is probable that his nagging concerns about clinical work were due to the fact that a career as a full-time medical scientist, divorced from any medical practice, was still a relative novelty in the United States in the 1890s.[20]

The Call to Johns Hopkins

Soon after his return from Europe to Ann Arbor in November 1892, Abel was contacted by William Osler, professor of medicine at Johns Hopkins, about the chair of pharmacology there. As discussed in chapter 1, the delay in the opening of the Johns Hopkins University School of Medicine had resulted in the abandonment of efforts to hire a pharmacologist. In 1890 a group of women established the Women's Fund Committee to raise the money needed to open the medical school. Largely due to a gift of about $300,000 from Mary Elizabeth Garrett, the daughter of the president of the Baltimore and Ohio Railroad, the committee was able to raise the necessary funds by the end of 1892. The money came with the condition that women must be admitted to the medical school as students on equal terms with men.[21]

At a meeting of the existing medical faculty of Johns Hopkins University on 12 January 1893, it was agreed that it would be desirable to appoint an instructor in pharmacology (among other subjects) before the scheduled opening of the medical school that fall. Abel's name must already have been in the minds of some of those present, because the very next day Osler wrote to him and asked: "On what terms could you be dislocated?" He added that he believed no one in the country had a better training in pharmacology than Abel.[22]

Several members of the medical faculty were already familiar with Abel's work. H. Newell Martin knew Abel personally from 1883, when Abel had worked in Martin's laboratory. At that time, Abel had also come into contact with Johns Hopkins President Daniel Coit Gilman and chemist Ira Remsen, though probably only casually. Abel had written to Martin, Gilman, and William Henry Welch, professor of pathology at Johns Hopkins, in 1888, when he was seeking an academic position, and outlined in detail his European studies and career plans.[23]

Both Osler and Welch were acquainted with Abel and respected his work. Welch had first met Abel in Ludwig's laboratory in Leipzig in 1885. In response to some reprints that Abel had sent him in 1892, Welch replied: "Your work is of a high order and so far as I know the only work in just the same direction which is done in this country." Osler and Abel had first met on a steamer bound for Europe in June 1892. Even before their first meeting, however, they had been in touch through correspondence, and Osler had expressed admiration for Abel's work.[24] Abel's long European apprenticeship also must have been impressive to the faculty of a university based so much on the Germanic model.

Thus, it is not surprising that Abel was the candidate of choice to be the first professor of pharmacology at Johns Hopkins. Because of delays in reaching agreement with Mary Garrett about the terms of her bequest, an official offer could not be made to Abel until March. After clarifying a few questions concerning salary and funding for laboratory help and supplies, Abel happily accepted the position. In a letter dated 2 March 1893, Osler had erroneously referred to a professorship of materia medica, and in his reply Abel requested that the title be changed to materia medica and pharmacology. It is clear (e.g., from the minutes of the Medical Faculty Advisory Board) that the title was intended to be pharmacology rather than materia medica, and that Osler had made a slip of the pen.[25] The Johns Hopkins medical faculty had recognized the importance of pharmacology over materia media a decade earlier when they attempted to hire Matthew Hay as professor of pharmacology.

In any case, when Abel arrived in Baltimore to take up his duties in September 1893, his title was professor of pharmacology. Later he stated that, as far as he could determine, this was the first chair in the country to carry the title *pharmacology*. The term had been used earlier as part of a combined title (e.g., chemistry, pharmacology, and materia medica), but Abel's chair at Hopkins was probably the first to carry the sole designation *pharmacology* and to use the word explicitly in the modern sense.[26]

Abel was also called upon to teach physiological chemistry in his first year, because no one had yet been appointed to that task, and his own pharmacology course was not to be taught until the second year of the medical curriculum. Physiological chemistry at Johns Hopkins remained nominally under his jurisdiction until 1908, when a separate department was created with Walter Jones as head. Jones had been hired as an assistant to Abel in 1896, and by 1899 had apparently taken over the major responsibility for the course.[27]

Before he arrived in Baltimore, Abel managed to fit in one more trip to Europe, returning to Berne in the summer of 1893 for further work in Drechsel's laboratory. In fact, he tried very hard to negotiate an opportunity to spend part of his first year at Johns Hopkins on leave in Europe. When his initial request to delay his arrival in Baltimore until 1 January 1884 was denied because it was felt that he should be on hand when the new medical school opened in the fall, Abel tried a different tactic. Because Abel's only responsibility during his first year was to teach the course in physiological chemistry, he proposed that he be allowed to get the course running smoothly, give the lectures, train the assistants, and then go abroad during the second semester (with the assistants presumably handling recitations and laboratory work in the course during this period). This request was also denied, however, as the medical faculty thought that it was important to have the principal instructors present during the entire first year.[28] Welch wrote to the undoubtedly disappointed Abel:

> I can not help feeling that after a man has had his training abroad, and yours has been most satisfactory and thorough, it is better for him to act independently on his own resources and develop his department. Remsen said that he has not felt that he could leave his duties at the university for a foreign sojourn since he began his connection with us. . . . I expect that you will give us a pharmacological department which will make it unnecessary to go abroad for good work in this line.[29]

John Abel left Ann Arbor in late May for Europe, and he apparently visited Schmiedeberg's laboratory in June. At the time, Arthur Robertson Cushny, a Scot who had received his medical degree from Aberdeen in 1889, was working in the pharmacological laboratory at Strassburg. Cushny had been at Berne, working with the physiologist Hugo Kronecker, in 1890 when Abel was in Nencki's laboratory. If they met at that time, they apparently did not get to know each other well. Now, however, perhaps on the advice of Schmiedeberg, Abel decided to write to Ann Arbor and recommend the young Scot for the chair of materia medica and therapeutics, which Abel had just vacated. The Board of Regents of the University of Michigan appointed Cushny to the chair in August, and he arrived in Ann Arbor in September to take up his duties.[30]

Arthur Cushny went on to become one of the leading pharmacologists of his generation. He remained at Michigan for twelve years, then returned to his native Britain in 1905, first to University College, London, and later to the University of Edinburgh, where he helped to establish pharmacology as a discipline in that country. In Cushny, Abel had found a colleague who would carry on the pharmacology program he had established at Michigan. Well trained in physiology, Cushny has spent two years as an assistant in Schmiedeberg's laboratory and, like Abel, represented the new experimental pharmacology rather than the old materia medica. A few years after his arrival in Ann Arbor, he published what can probably be considered to be the first modern textbook of pharmacology published in the United States, A Textbook of Pharmacology and Therapeutics (1899), a work that eventually went through thirteen editions.[31]

Cushny also began offering a laboratory course in pharmacology to the medical students on an optional basis. Although Abel had included experimental demonstrations in his lectures, during his relatively short stay at Michigan he did not provide the medical students with an opportunity for hands-on laboratory experience (except for advanced special students who might be allowed to undertake research with him). Shortly before Cushny left for England, this laboratory instruction was made a part of the required pharmacology course. The directions for the laboratory work had always been handed out in mimeographed form, but it seemed worthwhile to publish his laboratory manual in a more permanent form before Cushny departed. He and his assistant, Charles Edmunds (who succeeded him in the chair of materia medica and therapeutics at Ann Arbor) published their Laboratory Guide in Experimental Pharmacology in 1905. This little book was one of the earliest laboratory manuals published in experimental pharmacology.[32] An example of one of the experiments in the manual, demonstrating the pharmacological effects of the alkaloid veratrine, is as follows:

Inject 1 mg. of veratrine sulfate (1 cc. of 0.1% sol.) into a frog. Watch and describe the effects. Observe the awkwardness of its movements which appears in a few minutes. When the clumsiness is well developed locate the point at which the drug acts by removing the cerebrum, optic lobes, and finally destroying the spinal cord if the symptoms do not disappear earlier. Stimulate the sciatic plexus [a network of nerves supplying the limbs] with single shocks from the induction coil, comparing the results with those seen in a normal frog. Finally, stimulate the muscle directly, using single shocks. At what point does the drug act?[33]

This experiment was one of the simpler ones described in the manual. Students in the pharmacology course were expected to master such skills as anesthetizing rabbits and dogs and carrying out various surgical procedures on these anesthetized animals. Examples of such procedures are the insertion of cannulas into blood vessels, the trachea, and the bladder, and the dissecting out of nerves and glandular ducts. Participants in the course also learned to use standard instruments of the physiological and pharmacological laboratory, such as the kymograph for recording variations in blood pressure or other physiological functions. Students also indulged in self-experimentation, using a sphygmomanometer to measure their blood pressure after taking (by inhalation, ingestion, or injection) small quantities of such drugs as amyl nitrite, strychnine, atropine, and digitalin. Another example of human experimentation involved tobacco: "The effects of smoking upon the blood pressure may be tested upon a suitable individual; the most pronounced results will probably be obtained from inhaling the smoke from a 'strong' pipe or cigar."[34]

Abel's Career at Johns Hopkins

Abel arrived in Baltimore in mid-September of 1893, and his family joined him shortly thereafter. During his first year at Johns Hopkins, he taught only the physiological chemistry course. His pharmacology course was first offered to the medical students in the 1894–95 academic year, in the second year of the curriculum. The pharmacology course reflected Abel's belief in the importance of exposing students to the experimental method. Many of his lectures were accompanied by experimental demonstrations, as at Michigan. In addition, however, the course included a required laboratory component, with students working in groups of four. In an article on teaching pharmacology, Abel argued the case for laboratory work as follows:

Even if it is impossible for the student to perform more than a half-dozen experiments, this kind of work is too valuable to be omitted. Nowadays, when simple apparatus can be had at comparatively low cost, it is not a matter of great difficulty to give every four students out of a class of 75 a number of highly instructive experiments. These may be so arranged that the student himself learns the chief pharmacological facts involved, say, in the action of ether and chloroform, the diuretics and purgatives, atropin, morphin and chloral, or digitalis, the nitrites and other agents that have a pronounced action on the circulatory apparatus.[35]

Abel thus introduced significant participation in laboratory work as a part of the regular medical curriculum at a time when such teaching was the exception rather than the norm. It was in the same decade (the 1890s) that physiologists such as William Porter at Harvard and William Howell at Johns Hopkins began to include a significant amount of required laboratory work for medical students in their physiology courses. At the same time that Abel was writing the paper cited above, Porter was making it even easier and cheaper to obtain the necessary laboratory equipment for physiological and pharmacological work through the creation of his Harvard Physiological Apparatus Company.[36]

About 1907 the laboratory instruction was made optional (although experimental demonstrations were still included in the lecture course) because Abel believed that those medical students who did not take this laboratory course had ample opportunity to take other, related practical courses (such as pathology and physiology) involving vivisection experiments. Thereafter, he was able to accommodate only about half of the medical school class for laboratory instruction, and the course seems to have consistently reached its maximum limit. In fact, Paul Lamson, one of Abel's protégés who was at Johns Hopkins from 1914 to 1925, stated that students reportedly "bought" places in the class from each other for as much as twenty-five dollars.[37]

According to Lamson, the course was popular in spite of (or perhaps because of) the chaotic way in which it was operated, at least as of 1914 (by which time Abel had largely turned over the teaching of the course to assistants). Lamson described how Abel's two laboratory technicians would assemble all of the apparatus that they could find at the beginning of the semester and put it in a great heap on a table in the laboratory.

There was a worse jam at the apparatus table than at a bargain counter, members of the different groups shouting when they found a tambour or some other necessary object which all four members of their group were looking for. The scene around the table took on the aspects of the stock exchange in a panic, members of the different groups diving into the melee and signalling or shouting about the various parts of the apparatus which they sought. It was the custom to shave the dog before operating, but there was only one razor for the entire class. Elaborate methods of matching or tossing a penny for the razor were devised to see who could get it first. . . . These kymographs must have been out of date when they were bought at the opening of the medical school in 1893. It was impossible to make any of them run for any length of time, and you would hear a cheer from any group which managed to get a complete record of a single injection of a drug. The spirit of chance seemed to pervade the whole procedure in the laboratory.[38]

When Lamson's turn came to take charge of the course, he persuaded Abel to support his request to the dean to buy new equipment for the students, including a Harvard kymograph for each group. Lamson systematized the entire course procedure, insuring that each student group had everything it needed when the course began. He also arranged it so that the entire class could take the course. Everything ran in such an orderly fashion that one day Abel wandered into the laboratory and commented: "My goodness, Lamson, you certainly have ruined this course. The students used to have a good time here."[39]

Abel's greatest influence as a teacher was probably exerted more through his role as mentor to a generation of postgraduate pharmacology workers in his laboratory than through his medical school courses. He was not an especially good lecturer, and as his career progressed he turned more and more of his lecture duties over to his associates. Abel's laboratory, however, played a key role in the training of pharmacologists to fill the positions that were opening up in academic, industrial, and government institutions. In the last decade of the nineteenth century and the early part of the twentieth century, the Johns Hopkins pharmacology laboratory was one of the few American centers (and certainly the most prominent one) where an advanced student might receive training in the field. Among the prominent pharmacologists who worked with Abel in the period before the United States entered the First World War were Reid Hunt, the first pharmacologist hired by the federal government and later professor of pharmacology at Harvard; Arthur Loevenhart, first professor of pharmacology at the University of Wisconsin; Carl Voegtlin, head of the pharmacology division of the Public Health Service's Hygienic Laboratory and later head of the National Cancer Institute; Albert C. Crawford, professor of pharmacology at Stanford; H. G. Barbour, professor of pharmacology at Yale; Paul Lamson, professor of pharmacology at Vanderbilt; and E. K. Marshall, Jr., who eventually succeeded Abel as professor of pharmacology at Hopkins.[40]

These individuals did not receive their pharmacological training through formal graduate study. In fact, Abel was opposed to the establishment of a Ph.D. program in pharmacology, and such a program was not instituted at Hopkins until 1969, more than thirty years after his retirement. He believed that the ideal education for a pharmacologist was a solid grounding in chemistry and physics followed by training in medicine (preferably to the level of the M.D. degree). Those who went to work in Abel's laboratory usually had an advanced degree when they joined his staff. Hunt, Loevenhart, Crawford, Barbour, and Lamson, for example, had earned their M.D. degrees before entering Abel's laboratory (and Hunt had a Ph.D. in physiology as well). Voegtlin and Marshall came to Abel with doctorates in chemistry and some biomedical training.[41]

Thus Abel's protégés were essentially postdoctoral workers who assisted in the teaching of medical students and carried out research in his laboratory. Their training in pharmacology was achieved through working in an active research laboratory (although it did not have a large budget and was not particularly well equipped) and participating in teaching the subject. Abel apparently gave relatively little direction to his co-workers, except for those working directly with him on his own research projects, and they received no systematic training. Lamson noted that "men were simply turned loose and allowed to sink or swim," and that some "went through a great deal of mental anguish before finding a problem." He also added, however, that "they absorbed the spirit of the Professor, and after a very short time were working day and night."[42] Marshall described Abel's role as mentor as follows:

> Abel taught by example. He exercised a great influence on pupils, assistants and others who came into contact with him; he served unconsciously as a very effective catalyst for the research work of men

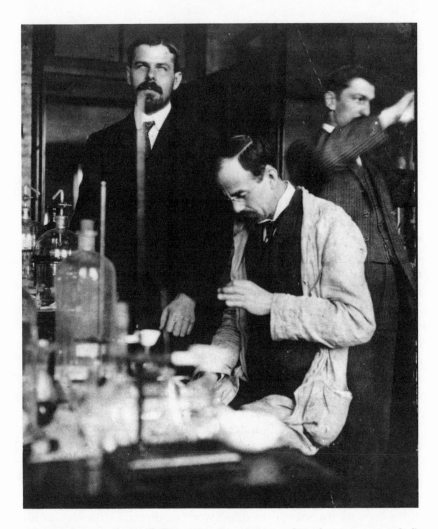

John Abel (seated), *Reid Hunt* (standing left), *and Walter Jones in Abel's laboratory at John Hopkins, 1901.*

Courtesy of the Alan Mason Chesney Medical Archives of the Johns Hopkins Medical Institutions.

working in his laboratory on their own problems. None failed to profit by his intense enthusiasm for his research, his youthful outlook on science, his tremendous optimism that the morrow would yield the coveted result, his fearlessness in engaging in difficult problems or in controversies and the simplicity of a very loveable man.[43]

E. M. K. Geiling, who worked with Abel throughout the 1920s, also claimed that Abel's greatest success as a teacher was in the laboratory, and that he taught largely by example, impressing his co-workers with his enthusiasm, industry, determination, and experimental technique.[44] Even serious accidents did not dampen Abel's enthusiasm for the laboratory. In 1900 Abel lost an eye in a laboratory explosion. In another explosion in 1902, Abel was overcome by amyl nitrate fumes and suffered an injury to his right hand from broken glass. While engaged in the research that led to the crystallization of insulin in 1926, Abel was hit by a car on his way home from the university and his leg was fractured. Abel, who was nearly seventy at the time, ignored medical advice and was back at work in the laboratory, on crutches and with his leg in a cast, two days after the accident.[45]

Abel tended not to discuss the details of his co-workers' research with them, and he barely glanced at the papers they wrote before sending them on for publication. Yet his former associates all stress the congenial and supportive atmosphere that he created for research in the laboratory, and the kind and friendly way in which he treated them. They looked upon Abel as a father figure, both in terms of their personal careers and in terms of the discipline of pharmacology as a whole.[46]

His former associates also consistently emphasize the importance of the daily lunch table discussions (which have acquired an almost legendary status in American pharmacology) on their scientific development. Typically everyone brought their own food to these daily luncheons, except for some items provided by general collection (such as tea and cookies) and occasional delicacies contributed by Mrs. Abel. The group would gather round an oilcloth-covered kitchen table, with Abel seated at the head on a chair and the others seated on laboratory stools. Roaches were such a problem in the laboratory that the group even tried putting the legs of the table in cans filled with kerosene to keep the insects from the food.

The luncheons were attended not only by those working in Abel's laboratory, but often by other members of the Hopkins faculty as well. In addition, visiting scientists sometimes joined the luncheon group. Much of the discussion centered around the latest developments in pharmacology, biochemistry, and related sciences, but the conversations could also range from the arts to sailing. The current research of the participants naturally received significant attention.[47] One of Abel's associates later commented that had he done nothing else in his years at Johns Hopkins but attend these luncheons, he "would

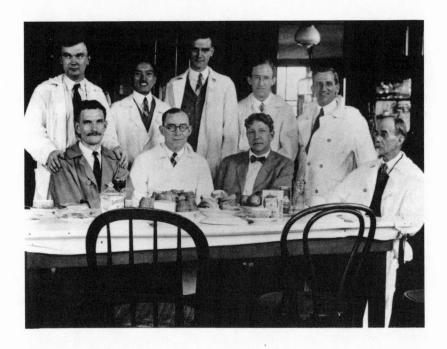

The lunch table group in Abel's laboratory at Johns Hopkins, about 1925.
Left to right, seated: C. A. Rouiller, E. M. K. Geiling, W. W. Ford, John
J. Abel; standing: J. V. Supniewski, Y. Ishikawa, Frederick Bell, Vincent
Vermooten, David Campbell.

Courtesy of the Alan Mason Chesney Medical Archives of the Johns Hopkins
Medical Institutions.

have acquired a liberal education and learned, in addition, the secrets
of successful graduate teaching."[48]

Not surprisingly, Abel was frequently consulted by academic colleagues at other institutions when they were seeking pharmacologists
for their staffs, as evidenced by the correspondence in the Abel Papers
at Johns Hopkins. Obviously a recommendation from Abel was a valuable asset to a young pharmacologist.

Abel as a Research Scientist

John Abel continued to carry out laboratory work with his own
hands throughout his career, never becoming solely a manager or

director of the research of others. Research was always his first love, and he devoted long hours to it. It is not my intent here to attempt to analyze in detail Abel's contributions to biomedical research, but rather to provide some idea of the topics that occupied his time and that of his associates over the years. He and his associates tackled challenging and significant problems, with an emphasis on the study of hormones.

When Abel arrived in Baltimore, he continued to work on some of his Ann Arbor investigations, such as the research on ethyl sulfide. In addition, he began efforts in new directions, the most important of which was to initiate research on the glandular products that were termed "hormones" (in 1905) by the English physiologist Ernest Henry Starling. His interest and training in physiological chemistry inclined him toward research on isolating the active principles of endocrine gland extracts. This was perhaps a natural extension of his work on the isolation of simpler organic substances, such as ethyl sulfide and carbamic acid, from natural sources. His first venture into the field of hormones, a subject which continued to hold his attention throughout most of his career, apparently involved an effort to obtain the active principle of thyroid gland extract. According to Abel, he abandoned this work in 1895 upon the announcement of Eugen Baumann's isolation of an organic compound of iodine from the gland.[49]

Abel turned to an attempt to isolate the active principle of the adrenal glands.[50] In 1895, George Oliver and Edward Schäfer, of University College, London, prepared an extract of the adrenal medulla that produced an immediate and dramatic rise in blood pressure when injected into experimental animals. A number of investigators, including Abel, almost immediately set about trying to isolate the active principle of Oliver and Schäfer's extract.

Using sheep adrenal glands provided by Armour and Company, Abel obtained a crystalline product that appeared to be the blood pressure-raising substance of Oliver and Schäfer's extract. He called it "epinephrin" and described it in a paper read before the Association of American Physicians on 6 May 1897 and published in the *Bulletin of the Johns Hopkins Hospital* later that same year.[51] Abel had obtained the active principle in the form of a crystalline benzoyl derivative, which he had then subjected to hydrolysis to remove the benzoyl groups. The residue that he obtained was physiologically very active, and Abel believed it to be the blood pressure-raising constituent of the adrenal gland, although in a state that was not quite pure. In two additional papers over the next two years, he expanded on this work and published a chemical formula for the compound.[52]

In 1901, Jokichi Takamine, a Japanese scientist who had settled in the United States, published the results of his own research on the adrenal substance, claiming that he had obtained the active principle in a pure, crystalline form.[53] Takamine argued that Abel's compound was either a modified substance or the benzoyl derivative which had withstood his hydrolysis treatment. Takamine gave a different chemical formula for his active principle, which he called "adrenalin." The compound was later marketed under the tradename of "Adrenalin" by Parke, Davis and Company, with whom Takamine had a working relationship. Parke-Davis chemist Thomas Aldrich, who also had been working on the problem, used a method differing slightly from that of Takamine to isolate a substance that was shown to be identical to adrenaline.[54] His chemical formula for the compound was somewhat different from Takamine's, and was later shown to be the correct one.

The discovery of epinephrine (the generic name preferred in the United States) or adrenaline, the first hormone to be isolated, was surrounded with controversy. There were disputes about the purity of the compounds isolated by the different investigators and about the correct formula and structure of the hormone. Because Takamine visited Abel's laboratory in 1899 or 1900, there were also suggestions in some quarters that he may have "borrowed" some of Abel's ideas. It is not clear, however, what Takamine would have learned in this way that he could not have obtained from Abel's published work, and depending upon the time of his visit, he may have been well on his way to his own success before meeting with Abel.

Eventually it was determined that Abel had isolated the monobenzoyl derivative of the hormone rather than the active principle itself. Takamine had actually isolated the hormone, although it was later shown that the natural product is itself a mixture of two substances, epinephrine and norepinephrine.[55]

In 1912 Abel isolated epinephrine in the toxic secretion of the parotid glands of the toad *Bufo aqua*. Other investigations in Abel's laboratory in the pre–World War I period included several chemotherapeutic studies and research on the pharmacological action of phthaleins and their derivatives. Abel's work with Leonard Rowntree on the phthaleins, published in the first volume of the pharmacology journal established by Abel (see chapter 5), serves as an example of a study of the pharmacological action of a particular substance or group of substances.

Abel and Rowntree set out to study the influence of chemical substitution in various parts of the molecule upon the pharmacological properties of the class of compounds known as phthaleins, keeping in mind the therapeutic goal of finding a serviceable hypodermic purgative. They compared the pharmacological (especially purgative) properties of a wide variety of phthalein derivatives. (The drugs were administered by various routes, but only hypodermic injection will be considered here.) The compounds were dissolved in olive oil, which was found to be a nonirritating solvent. In the experiments with dogs, the injections were made into the loose tissue at the back of the neck. The method for measuring the results were not exact—the investigators simply noting whether a laxative action could be recorded, by which they meant that *"the stools lost their hard and friable condition and became moist and pasty in consistence."* In this way, the tetrachlor derivative was found to be an effective laxative, whereas phenolphthalein and a number of other compounds gave poor results.

Since no toxic properties were observed, Abel and Rowntree (who was a clinician) next tried the tetrachlor derivative on a number of human patients suffering from chronic constipation, and were satisfied with the results. Rowntree had earlier tried the chlor derivative on himself at least once when he and Abel were still searching for the best solvent. Their paper also reported on the results of experiments on the excretion and absorption of the phthaleins.[56]

Abel's most important work in this period involved the development of his "vividiffusion" apparatus in 1913. The device allowed for the removal, by dialysis, of diffusible substances from the circulating blood of living animals. With this apparatus, Abel and his co-workers were able to demonstrate for the first time the presence of free amino acids in normal blood. Abel also recognized the clinical potential of the apparatus in cases of renal failure, although a functioning artificial kidney for clinical use was not developed until much later.

Although engaged in research on a variety of subjects, Abel retained his interest in problems of endocrinology, especially with respect to isolating hormones as pure chemical compounds. From about 1917 on, he devoted significant attention to an attempt to purify the active principle of the posterior pituitary gland. He never succeeded in this quest, however, in part handicapped by his firm but incorrect belief in the unitary nature of the pituitary hormone (there are actually several hormones produced by the posterior pituitary).[57]

In 1924 Abel turned his attention to insulin, the pancreatic extract prepared and introduced into therapy by Frederick Banting and Charles

Best and their colleagues at the University of Toronto in 1922.[58] The dramatic benefits of insulin in the treatment of diabetes were widely acclaimed, but it was recognized that the Toronto preparation contained many impurities and that it would be desirable to isolate the hormone in pure form. There was also disagreement about its chemical nature.

Abel embarked upon an attempt to isolate insulin at the suggestion of Arthur A. Noyes, professor of physical chemistry at the California Institute of Technology. In October 1924, Abel went to California with Eugene M. K. Geiling to spend four months getting started on the problem at the institute. This research occupied much of his time and energy for the next four years.

In November or December 1925, Abel first obtained insulin crystals, and he published a preliminary communication of his results in the February 1926 issue of the *Proceedings of the National Academy of Sciences*.[59] But the matter was far from settled. Abel soon began to encounter difficulty in reproducing the crystals by his original method. It took him about a year to repeat his success, using a somewhat modified technique.

In addition, Abel's claim that he had crystallized the pure hormone was challenged by some because his results suggested that his preparation was a protein. At the time, there was considerable skepticism about the ability of proteins to have the high degree of specific biological activity characteristic of a hormone. There was widespread acceptance of Richard Willstätter's view of enzymes, which held that the true enzyme was not a protein molecule, but an active chemical group associated with or held in colloidal state by a protein carrier. It was similarly argued that Abel's crystals were not the "real thing," but a protein carrier on which the true hormone was adsorbed. This objection was gradually overcome by the work of James B. Sumner, J. H. Northrop, and others in the late 1920s. Their work involved the crystallization of several enzymes which appeared to be homogeneous products whose biological activity depended upon their overall chemical structure, and not upon a distinct chemical group carried by the rest of the molecule. Assays of the potency of samples of insulin crystals produced in different laboratories, carried out in 1929, produced uniform results, providing further evidence for the chemical homogeneity of crystalline insulin.[60]

Research on insulin continued in Abel's laboratory for several more years, although he personally withdrew from the work and left it in the hands of his colleagues. Abel was typically more interested in the chemical challenge of isolating the hormone than in studying its physiological and pharmacological properties—topics that fell to co-workers such as Geiling to investigate. Chemical studies of insulin were also continued in the laboratory by a number of talented scientists, principally Hans Jensen, Oskar Wintersteiner, Vincent du Vigneaud and Earl A. Evans, Jr. Since he did not allow his name to be attached to scientific papers unless he had carried out at least some of the experimental work with his own hands, Abel does not appear as a coauthor of these later publications. The professor returned to his posterior pituitary research, a subject that continued to frustrate him. In the last years of his life, he turned his attention to a new subject for him, the study of tetanus toxin.[61]

From the point of view of Abel's place as a discipline builder, his laboratory was more important as a training ground for pharmacologists than for the individual discoveries that bear his name, many of which could be claimed as much by biochemistry as by pharmacology. His laboratory was the key institution in the education of the first generation of home-grown American pharmacologists. As pharmacology spread to other American medical schools, new research programs and laboratories for the training of more disciples were established by other practitioners of modern pharmacology, many of them protégés of John Jacob Abel.

CHAPTER FOUR

The Growth of Academic Pharmacology in the United States

The Reform of American Medical Education

Books by Ludmerer and by Rothstein have examined the reform of medical education that took place in the United States in the late nineteenth and early twentieth centuries.[1] This same period saw the rise of the modern university in this country, influenced by the German model. American colleges striving to become universities expanded their scope of interest to include the natural and social sciences as well as the classics, embraced professional education in fields such as law and medicine, and emphasized the discovery as well as the dissemination of knowledge. Medical education largely became incorporated into the universities, with academic medical schools increasingly replacing proprietary schools.

Medical curricula became longer and more rigorous. Requirements for admission to medical school were raised significantly, so that entering students were better prepared and more ambitious than previously. Teaching in medical schools became more demanding, and part-time practitioner-educators eventually came to be largely replaced by full-time instructors, at first in the scientific subjects, and later also in the clinical departments in many schools. Research became an important part of the medical school environment, as Americans worked to end their scientific dependence on Europe. The medical curriculum expanded to include new scientific subjects and clinical specialties, and laboratory work and clinical clerkships replaced or supplemented lectures in many areas.

Ludmerer has identified Harvard University, the University of Michigan, the University of Pennsylvania, and the Johns Hopkins University as the pioneers in the movement to reform medical education. In most cases this movement was led by faculty members who had studied abroad, especially in Germany, or had at least indirectly absorbed the Germanic tradition. Between the opening of the Johns Hopkins medical school in 1893 and the publication of the Flexner Report in 1910, the reforms initiated at these four institutions had spread to many other medical schools. Reform did not progress at a uniform pace, however, and there were great differences in the quality of medical schools at the time of the Flexner Report.[2]

Among the most significant of the changes in medical education was the important place of the new experimental sciences, such as physiology and bacteriology. Rothstein has pointed out that most medical schools first began to require laboratory courses in fields such as pathology, bacteriology, chemistry, and physiology in the 1890s.[3] Progress occurred unevenly in the different basic sciences. Ludmerer has argued that physiology was generally the best taught of the medical sciences, and that "pharmacology tended to be the weakest of the group, lagging behind the others despite the intense promotional efforts of John Jacob Abel at Johns Hopkins."[4]

Chapter 3 outlined how Abel introduced pharmacology into the curriculum at Michigan and at Johns Hopkins in the early 1890s. This chapter will examine the spread of the new experimental science to other American universities.[5]

The Dissemination of Pharmacology

Between Abel's arrival at Michigan in 1891 and the appearance of the Flexner Report in 1910, experimental pharmacology became an established field of study at a significant number of the nation's medical schools. Like the new biochemistry, which came to replace the traditional medical chemistry courses in the curriculum, pharmacology found a ready niche in the medical schools, in the slot formerly reserved for materia medica. Experimental pharmacology essentially replaced didactic materia medica, as the Germanic model, buttressed by Abel's example on this side of the Atlantic, came to prevail at reform-minded medical schools.

Robert Kohler has argued that the old medical chemists were not so much transformed into biochemists as they were replaced by the latter. He has pointed out that with both chemistry and materia medica, the differences between the old generation and the new were so great that the latter saw themselves as the pioneers of entirely new disciplines, biological chemistry and pharmacology.[6] Indeed, the new courses in pharmacology were generally taught by newly hired, laboratory-oriented faculty with some training in pharmacology, physiology, or physiological chemistry, rather than by those who had previously taught materia medica. At first, many of these individuals received at least part of their scientific training abroad, but in time more and more of them were trained at home in the laboratories of John Abel and other pioneers in American pharmacology. One of the new generation, Carl Alsberg, clearly articulated the opportunities open to him and his colleagues in 1908: "Chairs in [pharmacology] in our medical schools are held by elderly practitioners who lecture upon materia medica and therapeutics. Many of the chairs will soon be vacant and will be filled by professional pharmacologists. Adequately trained pharmacologists are, however, exceedingly rare in America at present."[7]

The first American medical school to truly make the transformation from materia medica to pharmacology after Michigan and Johns Hopkins was Western Reserve University. The transition began in 1894 with the appointment of John G. Spenzer as instructor in pharmacology and experimental therapeutics. Spenzer held an M.D. degree from Western Reserve and a Ph.D. degree from the University of Strassburg, where he spent some time studying with Schmiedeberg. He apparently began to offer laboratory instruction in pharmacology in 1894–95.[8]

Judging by the 1895–96 catalogue of the medical school, students were also subjected to a healthy dose of traditional materia medica from the professor of materia medica and therapeutics. In the discussion of materia medica and therapeutics, the catalogue notes that "illustrative lectures on animals" had been added to more clearly explain the physiological action of medicines, "thus bringing the teaching up to the most recent ideas." Schmiedeberg's book was one of the texts for the materia medica course. In addition, second-year students pursued pharmacological laboratory work as part of their materia medica course, and this laboratory work was continued in the third-year course on therapeutics.[9]

Spenzer's efforts at Western Reserve were relatively short-lived, however, as he left for another position at the end of the 1895–96 academic year. The expansion of laboratory work in pharmacology that was planned for the next year did not take place, and temporary arrangements were made for teaching the subject. In the spring of 1898, the teaching of pharmacology was assigned to Torald Sollmann, who had received his M.D. degree from Western Reserve in 1896 and was serving there as a demonstrator in physiology and histology. Sollmann instituted a course with a heavy laboratory component which was so successful that the faculty made him lecturer in pharmacology and eventually relieved him of his teaching duties in physiology. He was given funds to spend some time in Schmiedeberg's laboratory to further his knowledge of the subject. It almost appears that the Schmiedeberg stamp of approval was required to qualify one as a pharmacologist at the time.[10]

Torald Sollmann went on to become one of the influential forces in the early development of American pharmacology and is probably second only to Abel in reputation as a founder of the field in this country.[11] Sollmann was one of the founding members of the American Society for Pharmacology and Experimental Therapeutics and served as its second president (1913–15). For many years he also played an important role as a representative of pharmacology on such professional bodies as the Council on Pharmacy and Chemistry of the American Medical Association and the Committee on Revision of the United States Pharmacopeia. Sollmann's laboratory served as a training center for such future academic pharmacologists as Robert Hatcher (Cornell University), Paul Hanzlik (Stanford University), and Edgar Brown (University of Minnesota).[12] Sollmann's influence was also exerted through his widely used textbooks, the *Textbook of Pharmacology* (first published in 1901) and the *Manual of Pharmacology*, which was first published in 1917 and went through eight editions.[13]

Although the transition from materia medica to pharmacology began at several other medical schools (for example, see the discussions below of Northwestern, Pennsylvania, and Harvard) in the late nineteenth century, it was not until after 1900 that modern pharmacology became firmly established in American universities other than Johns Hopkins, Michigan, and Western Reserve. The pace of the transformation from materia medica to pharmacology significantly accelerated after the turn of the twentieth century. The new breed of experimental pharmacologists obtained positions in about ten more medical schools in the first decade of the new century. These appointments included five future presidents of the American Society for Pharmacology and Experimental Therapeutics: Robert Hatcher, Arthur Loevenhart, William deBerniere MacNider, Alfred Newton Richards, and George Wallace.

The three major medical schools in New York City, for example, all made the transition to modern pharmacology in the first decade of

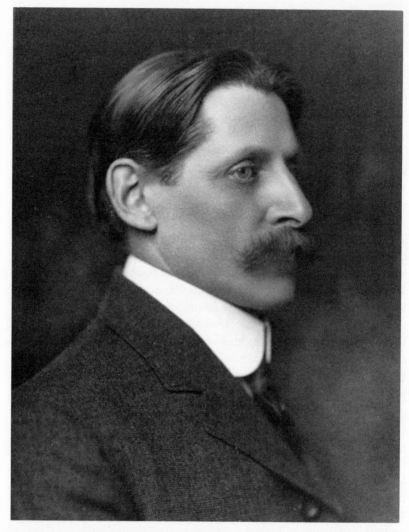

Torald Sollmann of Western Reserve University, one of the leading figures in the early development of American pharmacology.

Courtesy of the National Library of Medicine.

the twentieth century. The faculty appointed to these three pharmacology positions exemplified the training and outlook desired by medical schools seeking to replace didactic materia medica with the new pharmacological science. Both the Cornell University Medical School and the University and Bellevue Hospital Medical College of

New York University appointed M.D.'s who had apprenticed for several years in the laboratories of established pharmacologists. Robert Hatcher (Cornell) had served as an assistant to Sollmann at Western Reserve and George Wallace (New York University) as an assistant to Cushny at Michigan.[14]

Although Christian Herter, who was appointed to the chair of pharmacology at the College of Physicians and Surgeons of Columbia University in 1903, had not undergone a pharmacological apprenticeship like Hatcher and Wallace, he was well trained in experimental biomedical science. Herter had followed his M.D. degree with postgraduate laboratory studies at Johns Hopkins and in Switzerland, and then served as professor of pathological chemistry at the University and Bellevue Hospital Medical College.[15] Herter is generally associated more with biochemistry and pathology than with pharmacology, but the lines demarcating the various biomedical fields were not as clear at the turn of the century as they became later. John Abel, for example, is often counted by the biochemists as one of their own, and in fact Abel and Herter were the cofounders and coeditors of the *Journal of Biological Chemistry* in 1905 (see chapter 6). Herter was a proponent of the importance of laboratory research in medicine, and his appointment at Columbia was indicative of a conscious effort to move from materia medica to experimental pharmacology. In his history of the College of Physicians and Surgeons, published just a year after Herter joined the staff, F. S. Lee clearly recognized the change that had taken place at the college with this appointment:

> The time-honored term 'materia medica,' coupled with 'chemistry,' 'botany,' 'mineralogy,' 'institutes of medicine,' 'medical jurisprudence,' 'clinical medicine,' or 'therapeutics,' gave a title to a professor's chair in the College until 1903. In accordance with the growing importance of the study of the physiological action of drugs by exact experimental methods, it has now given place to the more timely title of pharmacology, and the change has carried with it the establishment of student laboratories of pharmacology and pharmacy.[16]

When Herter was appointed, he invited Alfred Newton Richards, who had received his Ph.D. in physiological chemistry from Columbia in 1901, to join his staff as an instructor. He especially wanted Richards to organize the laboratory course. At the time, Richards was working in Herter's laboratory on a Rockefeller Institute research scholarship.

Since neither Herter nor Richards was trained specifically in pharmacology, both of them spent some time working in Germany in 1903 to prepare for their new teaching responsibilities. Herter chose to visit the laboratories of Paul Ehrlich, the founder of modern chemotherapy, in Frankfurt and pharmacologist Hans Meyer in Marburg.

Richards meanwhile opted for the more time-honored pharmacological path of apprenticeship with Schmiedeberg. In the summer of 1903, Richards and George Wallace of New York University went to Strassburg, hoping to learn how to organize and conduct a student laboratory course in the subject. They were disappointed to find that there were no student laboratory exercises in Schmiedeberg's institute, but only didactic lectures and what they considered to be pedestrian research studies of advanced students.[17] It may be that Schmiedeberg, who was nearing the end of his career, was no longer the dynamic pharmacological leader that he had been earlier, or it may be that laboratory work and research were no longer so novel to Americans that they were easily impressed by German science. Richards and Wallace may also have been reacting to the situation described by Robert Kohler, namely, that laboratory work was available only to the select few in Germany, whereas American medical schools wanted to make it available to all students.[18] Although the Schmiedeberg name was still renowned enough to attract Richards and Wallace to his laboratory, the era of the pharmacological pilgrimage to Strassburg was clearly on the way out by this time.

Richards later became the first professor of modern pharmacology at the Northwestern University Medical School. Northwestern had introduced laboratory work in pharmacology as part of the required medical curriculum as early as 1896.[19] However, in 1907 J. H. Long of the Northwestern Medical School commented to Abel that he thought the work in pharmacology at his institution was out of date and the time had come for entirely new plans. Long admitted that Northwestern Medical School was more of a teaching than a research institution, and that the teaching load would be considerable. On Abel's recommendation, Northwestern hired Alfred Newton Richards as professor of pharmacology in 1908, clearly completing the transition to modern pharmacology with this move.[20]

The situation at the University of Wisconsin differed from other institutions in this chapter in that a medical school was not established in Madison until 1907. As was true of Johns Hopkins when Abel was appointed, the University of Wisconsin had no traditional medical curriculum to alter, and thus there was no transition to be made from materia medica to pharmacology. The medical school was founded in the midst of the period of reform of medical education and was able to establish a curriculum heavily based on laboratory science, including pharmacology.

Even before the opening of the medical school, the appointments of Charles Bardeen as professor of anatomy in 1904 and Joseph Erlanger as professor of physiology and physiological chemistry in 1906 made it clear that Wisconsin was determined to recruit well-trained medical scientists to its faculty. Both men had received their M.D. degrees from Johns Hopkins and had served as junior faculty in their specialties at their alma mater before being called to Madison.[21] Given Wisconsin's obvious predilection for Hopkins graduates, it is not surprising that they once again turned to Baltimore to fill the chair of pharmacology. For a third time Wisconsin raided the Johns Hopkins junior faculty, this time hiring Arthur S. Loevenhart as their professor of pharmacology. He had been an associate professor of pharmacology and physiological chemistry under Abel and possessed a medical degree from Johns Hopkins.[22]

The first medical school in the South to make the transition from materia medica to pharmacology was apparently Tulane University, with its appointment of John Taylor Halsey as professor of materia medica, therapeutics, and clinical medicine in 1904. The words "materia medica" in his title were changed to "pharmacology" in 1910. Halsey had studied pharmacology in Europe with Schmiedeberg and Meyer, and in 1914 he translated Meyer and Gottlieb's famous textbook of pharmacology into English.[23] In 1908 at the University of Virginia, John Augustine English Eyster, a Hopkins medical graduate with postgraduate training in Germany, was appointed professor of pharmacology, materia medica, and toxicology, replacing a man who had taught materia medica, hygiene, and medical jurisprudence at various times in his career.[24]

As the decade came to a close, the first appointment in pharmacology on the West Coast was made when Albert Crawford went to Stanford University in 1910. After obtaining his M.D. degree, Crawford worked as an assistant in Abel's laboratory from 1894 to 1900. He was working as a pharmacologist for the United States Department of Agriculture (see chapter 5) at the time he was hired for the Stanford position, largely through Abel's influence.[25] Stanford had earlier considered two other pharmacologists, Carl Voegtlin and Charles Edmunds, for the position, but was not able to obtain either of them.[26] Stanford President David Starr Jordan, incidentally, had an additional qualification for candidates besides their professional competence, as expressed in a letter to Abel: "One element in my attitude toward a professor is concerned with his relation to the general matter of temperance. I do not believe that the teachers of medicine ought to be users of alcoholics. I should not go so far as to oppose a good man for the use of tobacco. On the other hand, I would rather the men were not users of this drug."[27]

When Abraham Flexner's report on medical education appeared in 1910, pharmacology was an established discipline at a significant number of American medical schools, especially at the better universities. The institutions in Flexner's "first division," those that required two years of college work prior to admission to the medical school, generally had four separate laboratories, one of which was pharmacology. There were only sixteen medical schools in this group, however, with another nine scheduled to join their ranks shortly. Some of the better schools in the "second division" (requiring graduation from high school for admission) had pharmacology laboratories, but the great majority of institutions in this category did not. As for the "third division" schools, which Flexner considered to be "basely mercenary," the report dismissed their laboratory teaching as "hardly more than make-believe."[28]

Flexner himself emphasized that the science of pharmacology should form the basis for rational therapeutics and that medical students should be exposed to laboratory work in the subject with experimental animals. He also referred to materia medica as a subject "now much shrunken." On the other hand, it is obvious from the report that many medical schools still did not have pharmacological laboratory facilities and courses, and depended heavily on didactic lectures (which may have included more of the traditional materia medica than Flexner would have wished) to teach pharmacology. In 1910 the transition from materia medica to pharmacology was well underway, but by no means completed.[29] A detailed examination of the medical schools at Pennsylvania, Harvard, and North Carolina provides a more concrete understanding of the process of transition.

The University of Pennsylvania

As discussed in chapter 1, the University of Pennsylvania School of Medicine had already begun the transition to modern pharmacology in the late nineteenth century with the appointment of Horatio C Wood as professor of materia medica, pharmacy, and general therapeutics. Wood also served as clinical professor of nervous diseases. Although still essentially a part of the "old guard" of materia medica teachers rather than the new breed of pharmacologists, Wood was probably the most forward-looking of the group in his approach to the subject; for one thing, he engaged in experimental pharmacological research.

Before 1898 instruction in materia medica and therapeutics at Pennsylvania appears to have consisted entirely of lectures. Advanced studies, however, were encouraged to consider pursuing laboratory research in some specialized area. One of their options was to work under the direction of Wood in the laboratory of experimental therapeutics, "furnished with all the apparatus and instruments necessary for the study of the physiological action of medicines." Undoubtedly, relatively few students were exposed to pharmacological experimentation.[30]

In November 1897, Wood proposed introducing an elective course on experimental pharmacology into the curriculum. He also recommended that weekly demonstrations in pharmacology be given to all third-year medical students and requested the establishment of a position of demonstrator to handle the teaching. That there was still some uncertainty about the new subject and its relationship to therapeutics (and perhaps also about the relationship of laboratory science to practical medicine) is reflected in the fact that there was significant discussion among the faculty over the title of the demonstrator and the course. Should the course title be "experimental therapeutics" or "experimental pharmacology"? Wood also proposed the title of "practical pharmacology," which suggests that there might have been some concern that instruction in the subject not to be too theoretical. Wood seems not to have held strong views about the name, and in the end the title "pharmacodynamics" was given to both the demonstrator and the course. The committee that had been appointed to make a recommendation on the matter also apparently considered changing the title of Wood's chair as well, but decided to leave that as it was.[31]

Wood's son, Horatio C. Wood, Jr., was appointed to the new post, and "Demonstrations in Pharmacodynamics" first appeared as a third-year medical course in the 1898–99 catalogue. The younger Wood had received his medical degree from Pennsylvania in 1896, and then studied in Berne, Switzerland, before joining the faculty at his alma mater. He served in the position of demonstrator for the next nine years. His role was expanded in the 1901–2 academic year, when he took over one of the two weekly lectures in his father's therapeutics course to cover the physiological action of drugs. Two years later, a three-hour, one-semester pharmacology laboratory course was introduced at Pennsylvania, so that students could carry out "hands-on" laboratory exercises to supplement the knowledge of experimental techniques learned via demonstrations.[32]

Wood was probably grooming his son to be his successor, but if that was indeed his plan, he was destined to be disappointed. In 1904 the medical faculty proposed the creation of a position of assistant professor of pharmacology, with the younger Wood recommended as the candidate to fill it. The university's Board of Trustees was slow to act on the proposal, and eventually turned it down in March 1905 on the recommendation of its Committee on the Department of Medicine, which believed that the time had not yet come for such a move. In that same month, the senior Wood wrote to Abel to request that he send a letter of recommendation to Michigan on his son's behalf. Arthur Cushny had announced his intention to leave Michigan, thus vacating the chair of pharmacology there, and Wood hoped to secure the post for his son. He explained to Abel that constant friction between himself and the provost of the university, Charles Harrison, had made the position of the two Woods "anything but restful." However, Wood did not get the Michigan position.[33]

In 1906 failing health forced Wood, Sr., to retire from his chair of materia medica, pharmacology, and general therapeutics. At a meeting of the medical faculty on 17 December 1906, there was an extended discussion of what should be done with the chair. The principal question involved was this: should Wood's successor continue to have such broad duties, or would it be better to create two chairs, one in pharmacology and one in applied therapeutics? Alternatively, it was suggested that the teaching of therapeutics be delegated to those already engaged in teaching clinical medicine, thus avoiding the need to create a separate chair.

There seems to have been widespread agreement on the need to establish a chair of pharmacology and to fill it with someone, in the words of professor of ophthalmology George de Schweinitz, "who would probably possess the title of Pharmacologist, and who is not a practicing physician and therefore not dependent upon practice for his support." De Schweinitz went on to state that the pharmacologist should have the same relation to his chair as the professor of physiology does to his. David Edsall, assistant professor of medicine, also expressed the view that "in the present trend of events in this and other countries, it seems to me very advisable to have a Professor of Pharmacology (whatever is done with the rest of the Chair) who shall be chiefly a student of Pharmacology, and who shall teach pharmacological methods as is being done in most of the advanced institutions elsewhere." Dr. Philip Hawk, a physiological chemist, agreed that all of the leading medical schools were making more of the study of pharmacology than in the past, and he pointed out that a chair in the subject had been established at Columbia several years earlier. The faculty also favored the idea of having a chair of applied therapeutics and unanimously voted to recommend the creation of two chairs.[34]

In spite of Pennsylvania's excellent reputation as a medical school, Provost Harrison was concerned that the university was lagging behind its rivals in the experimental medical sciences, especially after the departure of Simon Flexner in 1903. He and his nephew, Charles Harrison Frazier, dean of the medical school, were making efforts to bring in new blood, and especially faculty with strong research orientations, to strengthen the school.[35] They no doubt welcomed the effort to appoint a modern experimental pharmacologist to a chair. Pennsylvania set its sights high and approached the widely respected Arthur Cushny, who had just recently returned to his native Britain to accept a chair of pharmacology at the University of London. Cushny declined.[36]

Perhaps the failure to attract a pharmacologist of the calibre of Cushny led Pennsylvania to abandon its plan to establish separate chairs of pharmacology and therapeutics. Instead, in 1907 one of its own faculty, David Linn Edsall, was appointed to a combined chair of therapeutics and pharmacology (note that therapeutics came first in the title). Just about two years after he was denied an assistant professorship, Horatio C. Wood, Jr., was made associate professor of pharmacology, perhaps as a consolation for not obtaining his father's chair. Wood continued to handle the lectures and laboratory work in pharmacology, while Edsall taught the therapeutics course.[37] In 1908 Edsall outlined the division of responsibilities between Wood and himself in a letter to Sollmann:

I would say that laboratory work and demonstrations in pharmacology are given the students under Dr. Wood; and that he also gives, for half the year, a course of lectures that discuss from a descriptive standpoint the pharmacological effects of the drugs that have a somewhat important and complex physiological action, pointing out in a general way the directions in which these drugs may be employed clinically in accordance with their physiological action. My own systematic discussions of the uses of the drugs comes twice a week in the last half of the year; and they consist in discussing drugs after the manner in which a clinician who tries to be accurate in his use of such remedies employs them. That is, I take up the types of conditions that we meet with clinically. . . . I then, with each condition that I am discussing, take up the whole group of drugs that are really important in connection with the condition."[38]

Although Wood seems to have been well grounded in pharmacology and was one of the founding members of the American Society for Pharmacology and Experimental Therapeutics, he never became a leader in the field. As for Edsall, though he was a strong proponent of experimental medicine and the reform of medical education, he was not a pharmacologist. Soon after moving to the chair of medicine in 1910, he left Philadelphia, spending a brief period at Washington University in St. Louis before moving on to Harvard University, where he had a distinguished career, serving for many years as dean of the medical school.[39]

With the vacancy created by Edsall's move to the chair of medicine, Pennsylvania this time took the opportunity to create a separate chair of pharmacology, divorced from therapeutics. The Board of Trustees acted on 7 June 1910 to appoint A. N. Richards to the position. The course in therapeutics, meanwhile, was taken over by the Department of Medicine and taught by Edsall and then his successor.[40] Richards had previously taught pharmacology with Herter at Columbia and served as professor of the subject at Northwestern. In Richards, Pennsylvania had acquired someone who would go on to become one of America's most prominent pharmacologists, and thus assured itself a significant role in the further development of the discipline in America. Richards also became a major figure in the administration of the University of Pennsylvania, serving as Vice-President for Medical Affairs from 1938 to 1948, and in national science policy, serving as chairman of the Committee on Medical Research from 1941 through 1946.[41]

As for Horatio C. Wood, Jr., the appointment of Richards meant that he had been passed over for a second time for the chair of pharmacology. Undoubtedly discouraged about his prospects at Pennsylvania, he moved to the Medico-Chirurgical College of Philadelphia as professor of pharmacology and therapeutics in 1910. He held this position until the institution was merged with the University of Pennsylvania School of Medicine in 1917. Wood thus found himself back at his alma mater, where he played only a secondary role in pharmacology in the shadow of his better-known colleague Richards.[42]

Harvard University

As with other American medical schools, instruction in materia medica was included in the medical curriculum at Harvard from the founding of the school in 1782. At first, the professorship of materia medica was combined with chemistry, but later materia medica was given its own chair. A history of the Harvard Medical School published in 1906 notes that in the earlier part of the institution's history "very little was known about the action of drugs so that most of the time was spent in studying and teaching their physical and chemical properties and botanical history." The authors claim that there is no evidence of any attempt to teach pharmacology in an experimental way before 1871, but that some beginning was made in this area with the appointment of Dr. Robert T. Edes as assistant professor of materia medica in that year.[43]

The beginning in pharmacology made by Edes appears to have been a very limited one. The description of the materia medica course in the 1871–72 catalogue stated that it was taught by recitations, "as this mode of instruction is best adapted for imparting that practical knowledge of drugs and their properties, which can only be obtained from the examination of specimens and pharmaceutical preparations, of which there is an extensive collection." Although this course apparently followed the typical didactic lines for the subject, the catalogue went on to add that "*therapeutics, or the physiological action of drugs and their application to disease, will be taught in the third year by lectures.*" There is no mention of experimental demonstration or laboratory work, and it is not clear how much pharmacology per se, as opposed to traditional therapeutics, was covered in the lecture course.[44]

Whatever changes there were in the teaching of materia medica were probably connected with the reform of medical education that was just beginning at Harvard under President Charles Eliot. The length of the academic year was increased, admission criteria and academic standards at the medical school were raised, and laboratory science was given greater prominence. In 1871, for example, Henry Pickering Bowditch, one of the founders of American physiology, joined the faculty and established a physiological laboratory. It was to be some time, however, before pharmacology achieved the level of physiology at Harvard.[45]

In 1884 the next stage in the transition from materia medica to pharmacology appears to have occurred, when the course in therapeutics was divided into two series of lectures—once a week on "clinical therapeutics" and twice a week on "experimental therapeutics." Joseph W. Warren, instructor in experimental therapeutics and assistant in physiology, taught the latter course. Francis H. Williams, instructor in materia medica, taught the course in that subject.

In 1885 Williams's title was changed to instructor in materia medica and therapeutics, and he was placed in charge of the department. Over the next few years, Williams moved Harvard further along the road of experimental pharmacology.[46] Williams, the son of the famous Harvard ophthalmologist Henry Willard Williams, received his medical degree from Harvard in 1877. He then spent two years studying in Europe, including a stint in Schmiedeberg's laboratory, and hence was familiar with the German tradition of experimental pharmacology. After several years in the private practice of medicine in Boston, he joined the Harvard faculty in 1884.[47]

Williams introduced demonstrations into the therapeutics course, although the nature of these demonstrations is not clear and they apparently did not involve student participation. It seems likely, given Williams' training, that he demonstrated the physiological effects of drugs on experimental animals. When he was trying to recruit Abel to join him as an assistant in 1890, he commented to Mary Abel that pharmacology had been the subject that he had studied most thoroughly in Europe, but since there were no openings in this field in the United States, he had accepted the materia medica and therapeutics position at Harvard. He also expressed to her the hope that having an assistant like Abel would enable him to initiate an active experimental research program in pharmacology and therapeutics.[48]

Abel went to Ann Arbor instead of Boston, of course, and Williams left Harvard in 1891 for an appointment on the medical staff of the Boston City Hospital. Within a few weeks after Roentgen's discovery of x-rays in December 1895, Williams had become so interested in the new discovery that he was using x-rays to study cases of pulmonary tuberculosis and other thoracic lesions. He essentially abandoned his interest in pharmacology and became an American pioneer in the fields of roentgenology and radium therapy. Under Williams's successor, Charles Harrington, opportunities were provided for a limited number of undergraduate medical students to elect to undertake original research (probably some form of supervised independent study) in a laboratory of experimental pharmacology and therapeutics. According to the catalogue, this work offered an opportunity "for practical training and instruction in the methods and uses of the special apparatus employed in determining the toxic and physiological action of drugs and their practical values as remedies."[49]

Franz Pfaff, who joined the faculty as an instructor in pharmacology in 1895 and rose to the rank of full professor of pharmacology and therapeutics in 1905, provided the bridge to the modern era of pharmacology at Harvard that began in 1913. Pfaff received a Ph.D. from the University of Zürich, apparently in chemistry, and later an M.D. from Strassburg, where he worked with Schmiedeberg. He also did postgraduate work in medicine in London, and then served for three years as director of the chemistry laboratory in the province of Amazonia in Brazil, where he studied the medicinal plants of the region.[50] In 1902 Pfaff gave the first course at Harvard that actually bore the title of pharmacology rather than materia medica or therapeutics. In 1910 he introduced an elective course in experimental pharmacology open to fourth-year medical and postgraduate students.[51]

Although Pfaff had the necessary credentials to be one of the new breed of pharmacologists, having been a pupil of Schmiedeberg, he was always on the fringe of the active pharmacological community. He published a reasonable number of papers early in his career, especially based on the work he did in Brazil, but soon after his arrival at Harvard his research productivity declined. A search of *Index Medicus* reveals only a handful of research papers by Pfaff after 1898, and none of special significance.[52]

Pfaff's relatively low standing among his colleagues, especially considering his position at one of the country's most prestigious universities, is reflected in the discussions concerning whether he should be asked to join the editorial board of the *Journal of Pharmacology and Experimental Therapeutics* when it was founded in 1909. Arthur Loevenhart was opposed to placing Pfaff on the board, arguing that he had enjoyed as fine an opportunity to pursue work in the field as any man in the country, but had done nothing. In fact, Loevenhart argued that Pfaff had actually impeded the progress of pharmacology in the United States by his lack of research activity, expressing the view to Abel that "if the Harvard chair had been filled by a worker so that your chair had not stood alone pharmacology would not have waited until 1909 to emancipate itself." Torald Sollmann was willing to go either way on the question, but leaned toward placing Pfaff on the board, especially "if it could be delicately suggested to Pfaff" that he was "expected to be of more active assistance to Pharmacology." If part of Abel's plan in appointing members to the board was to help insure that papers from their laboratories would be submitted to the journal, Sollmann ventured the opinion that this would not matter in Pfaff's case because "there are none of Pfaff's to get." In the end, Abel did invite Pfaff to join the board, probably because of Pfaff's position and seniority.[53]

When Pfaff decided to retire as of 1 February 1913, largely for health reasons, a committee was established to recommend a successor. The committee consisted of four distinguished medical scientists: Walter Cannon (professor of physiology), David Edsall (professor of clinical medicine), Otto Folin (professor of biochemistry) and Milton Rosenau (professor of preventive medicine and hygiene). It seems clear that the group recognized that Harvard had not yet done justice to this field as it had to other biomedical sciences, because, in a letter to the dean of the medical school, Cannon referred to the question of "organizing" a department of pharmacology and to the expenses needed to operate a first-class department in the field. He also noted that a salary of at least $5,000 would probably be needed to recruit a pharmacologist since the number available was "extremely meagre."

Pfaff apparently recommended that Harvard try to induce Abel to accept the position. The committee considered this suggestion, but concluded that "the calling of another man from Baltimore would be rather brazen and furthermore that Abel is arriving at an age at which productive scholarship is not likely to be so abundant as it has been in the past." Their first choice for the position was Abel-protégé Reid Hunt, but Cannon noted that Harvard would probably have to match the salary of $6,000 that he earned at the Hygienic Laboratory of the United States Public Health Service (see chapter 5). He also noted that Hunt was known to be a poor teacher, and that if he were brought to Harvard it would have to be for his abilities as a scientific investigator, with teaching responsibilities largely handled by subordinates.[54]

In 1913 Harvard did indeed recruit Hunt as professor of pharmacology, marking the beginning of the "modern era of pharmacology" at Harvard, as noted by Beecher and Altschule in their history of medicine at the university. With Hunt's arrival, the name of the department was finally listed as "pharmacology" rather than "materia medica and therapeutics" in the university's catalogue. The pharmacology department itself considers its date of establishment to be 1913, when Hunt was appointed.[55]

Hunt was an influential and widely respected figure in American pharmacology. He was superbly trained to fill the role of a modern experimental pharmacologist. He held both a Ph.D. in physiology from Johns Hopkins University and an M.D. from the College of Physicians and Surgeons in Baltimore, and he had pursued medical studies at the University of Bonn, where he first acquired an interest in pharmacology under Karl Binz. Hunt was an assistant and then an associate professor of pharmacology in Abel's department from 1898 to 1904, making two trips during that time to work for some months in the laboratory of Paul Ehrlich in Germany. In 1904 he became chief of the Hygienic Laboratory's Division of Pharmacology.

Although Hunt made his greatest research contributions before coming to Harvard, he remained an active investigator until his retirement from the Harvard chair in 1936. He was also extremely active in a professional capacity in the pharmacological field. Hunt served as the first secretary, and then later as president, of the American Society for Pharmacology and Experimental Therapeutics; as a member of the American Medical Association's Council on Pharmacy and Chemistry for thirty years; and as president of the Committee on Revision of the United States Pharmacopeia for ten years.[56]

University of North Carolina

Although there was a short-lived school of medicine at the University of North Carolina from 1879–85, a continuous tradition of medical education at the institution did not begin until 1890. The medical department that opened in Chapel Hill in September of that year initially offered only a one-year curriculum, and was designed to be preparatory to a "diploma granting college." Dr. Richard Whitehead, who had received his medical degree from the University of Virginia in 1887, headed the department and also served as professor of anatomy, physiology, and materia medica. Whitehead's real interest was in anatomy, and when the department expanded to a two-year curriculum and increased its faculty in 1896, he became professor of anatomy and pathology. Charles Magnum, an 1894 graduate of Jefferson Medical College who had earlier completed the one-year medical course at North Carolina, was hired as professor of physiology and materia medica.[57]

The description in the 1890 medical school catalogue of the materia medica course taught by Magnum indicates that the course followed the traditional didactic approach to the subject: "This constitutes the study of the geographical and botanical sources of drugs, their physiological and toxic effects, and, to a less extent, the indications for their rational use. Opportunities will be given the student to familiarize himself with many of the crude drugs and their preparations."[58]

In 1902 the university opened a clinical branch of the medical school in Raleigh, due to the lack of facilities for clinical teaching in Chapel Hill. The opening of this department meant that students could now earn the M.D. degree from the University of North Carolina by completing their preclinical studies in Chapel Hill and their clinical work in Raleigh. The first student to register for the new program in Raleigh was William deBerniere MacNider, the university's future professor of pharmacology. A native of Chapel Hill, MacNider had received his undergraduate degree there and then enrolled in the medical school. During his preclinical years in Chapel Hill, he served as an assistant in anatomy. MacNider was in the first graduating class at Raleigh in 1903, and remained there as a demonstrator in clinical pathology and diagnosis for the next two years.[59]

In 1905 Whitehead left to go to the University of Virginia, and Isaac Manning, who had joined the faculty as professor of physiology and bacteriology in 1901, was appointed as his successor as dean of the medical school. University President Francis Venable, a chemist by training, decided to use the occasion of Whitehead's departure to reorganize the teaching responsibilities and expand the faculty from three to five. He seems to have been particularly concerned that the loss of Whitehead, the founding dean, would lead to fears that there would be a weakening of the medical department, and he took steps to demonstrate his support of the program.[60]

Since Whitehead did not resign until July, Venable was in a poor position to recruit faculty for the fall. Richard Henry Lewis, professor of diseases of the eye and ear at the Raleigh branch, had strong views about what should be done at Chapel Hill and contacted Venable, who welcomed his advice. Lewis thought highly of MacNider, and Venable gave him the approval to try to recruit the young physician to Chapel Hill. Unlike the well-established medical schools at Pennsylvania and Harvard, where a conscious decision was made to hire a bona fide pharmacologist, the advent of modern pharmacology at North Carolina came about in a much less direct way.[61]

Although he was to go on to become a leader in the field, MacNider did not have the training or expertise in pharmacology that other rising young stars of the science, such as Arthur Loevenhart or Reid Hunt, had at the time they assumed professorships in the subject. Apparently neither Venable nor Lewis decided to recruit MacNider specifically as a pharmacologist. Rather, they were impressed by MacNider's overall ability at a time when they were desperately trying to find qualified teachers for the rapidly approaching academic year. MacNider was asked about his preferences for teaching. He indicated that he preferred to teach a subject that was closer to practical than to theoretical medicine, and materia medica seemed to him to come closest to fulfilling that criterion of all the subjects taught in the preclinical medical program at Chapel Hill.[62]

Venable talked to Charles Magnum, who was willing to devote himself entirely to anatomy and to turn materia medica over to MacNider, of whom he thought highly. Magnum was therefore made professor of anatomy, succeeding Whitehead in this capacity. In 1905 MacNider joined the Chapel Hill faculty, with the title of professor of pharmacology and bacteriology. Although *bacteriology* was soon dropped from his title, it appears that MacNider continued to teach the course for some time. Presumably he was assigned this latter subject as well so that Manning, who was to assume the deanship, could be relieved of this teaching responsibility, although he continued as professor of physiology. These developments at North Carolina are indicative of the lack of fixed qualifications for faculty positions in the biomedical sciences at the turn of the century in American medical schools, especially in those that were not of the first rank.[63]

Although MacNider had no specific training in pharmacology, it seems clear that he and his colleagues recognized the need to replace materia medica with modern experimental pharmacology. Aside from the change in name of the professorship, the report of Dean Manning for 1905 emphasized the need to provide a laboratory for proper instruction in pharmacology. In fact, Manning emphasized that the "new curriculum" demanded a greater amount of laboratory training in general, and he complained that the present laboratory facilities were inadequate. MacNider added pharmacology to materia medica in the title of the course, supplemented the lectures with laboratory work (replacing recitations and demonstrations), and soon switched from the more traditional materia medica textbooks to Sollmann's more modern pharmacological text.[64]

Because MacNider recognized that he lacked proper training in the subject in which he now possessed a chair, he decided to spend part of the summer of 1906 at Rush Medical College in the laboratory of physiologist and pharmacologist Samuel A. Mathews, one of the founding members of the American Society for Pharmacology and Experimental Therapeutics. In the two subsequent summers, he worked in Torald Sollmann's laboratory at Western Reserve University.[65]

In a 1909 article in the *Southern Medical Journal*, MacNider made the case for the teaching of pharmacology even in smaller medical schools. He explained how such a course, including laboratory work, could be given at a very modest cost. Obtaining the dogs needed for the experimental work was not a problem, according to MacNider: "In the larger cities it is fairly easy to obtain the dogs necessary for this work from 'dog catchers' and the city pound. At institutions located in small towns this source of supply is wanting. It is astonishing how rapidly dogs develop the habit of sucking eggs and catching chickens when it has become known in the community that they are selling at fifty to seventy-five cents a head."[66]

MacNider eventually became one of the more widely respected pharmacologists of his generation, serving as president of the national society in the period 1933–35 and carrying out important research on the physiology, pathology, and pharmacology of the kidney. He also served as dean of the medical school at North Carolina from 1937 to 1940.

Pharmacology in Schools of Pharmacy

The early development of professional pharmacology in the United States was centered in the medical school environment. Since physicians are not the only health professionals requiring a knowledge of the effects of medicinal substances, it is not surprising that courses in pharmacology eventually also found their way into the curricula of schools of dentistry, nursing, veterinary medicine, and pharmacy. The subject has not been significantly developed in colleges of arts and

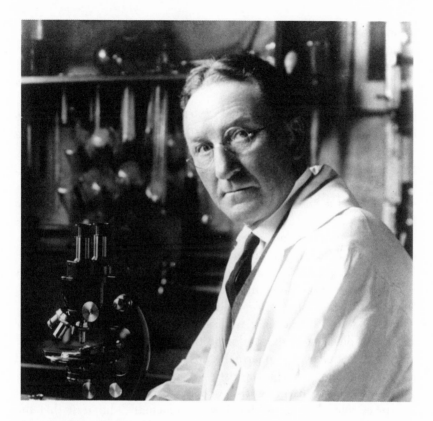

Pharmacologist William deBerniere MacNider in his laboratory at the University of North Carolina at Chapel Hill in 1946.

Courtesy of the National Library of Medicine.

sciences, remaining instead firmly within the sphere of the health professions schools.

For most of these schools, courses in pharmacology performed a service function and were often taught by medical school faculty members. In more recent times, however, schools of pharmacy and of veterinary medicine, at least, have come to join medical schools as respectable academic homes for research-oriented pharmacologists. One measure of this trend is found in a 1988 directory of graduate programs in pharmacology, which listed 38 such programs in colleges of pharmacy and 18 in schools of veterinary medicine (as opposed to 132 in medical schools) in the United States.[67]

Pharmacology has gained an especially prominent position within the pharmacy school curriculum as pharmaceutical education has evolved toward training the pharmacist to be an expert on drugs rather than a compounder of medicines. The clinical pharmacy movement that began in the 1960s, and gained headway in the decades that followed, has led some pharmaceutical educators to refer to pharmacology as "the focus of the curriculum thrust" toward biological science and "the keystone course in the curriculum."[68] These recent developments are beyond the scope of this book, but the roots of pharmacology as a subject in the pharmacy curriculum go back to the nineteenth century. It therefore seems worthwhile to at least briefly examine the evolution of the field in American schools of pharmacy as an example of the establishment of the discipline in an academic setting other than the medical school.[69]

The standard pharmacy school curriculum of the nineteenth century included a course in materia medica, a subject of great practical interest to the pharmacist of the period. These materia medica courses covered much of the same material as those taught in medical schools: the origins, constituents, preparations, and therapeutic uses of drugs. As pharmacists increasingly replaced physicians as teachers of the subject in pharmacy schools during the course of the century, more emphasis was placed on pharmacognosy (i.e., the natural history and physical and chemical characteristics of crude drugs) and less on therapeutics. Several pharmaceutical educators stressed that the needs of pharmacy and medical students were sufficiently different that the materia medica courses aimed at each must also be different. In particular, there was a belief that pharmacy students did not require an intimate knowledge of the physiological and therapeutic action of drugs.[70]

Thus it should not be surprising to find that pharmacy schools were generally slow to abandon their materia medica courses for the new pharmacology when the latter subject began to enter the medical schools. A few far-sighted educators did manage to introduce the teaching of pharmacology in the pharmacy school environment, most notably at the University of Michigan and the University of Nebraska.

Since its founding in 1868, under the leadership of its dean, physician-chemist Albert Prescott, the University of Michigan School of Pharmacy had pioneered in the development of a basic science–oriented curriculum with a significant laboratory component. Throughout the 1880s, the materia medica course in the pharmacy curriculum was taught by faculty in the medical school and included "lectures on the physiological action of drugs." In 1891, with the arrival of John Abel, the catalogue listed a lecture course (including demonstrations) in

"Pharmacology and Therapeutics," in addition to the materia medica class. During his first year at Michigan, Abel's pharmacology course was composed of third-year medical students, dental students, and pharmacy students. Apparently Abel concluded that the dental and pharmacy students did not possess sufficient knowledge of physiology and medicine for the course, because in 1892 the pharmacology course was listed in the pharmacy school catalogue as an elective rather than as a requirement, and may have required Abel's permission for enrollment.

The 1895 pharmacy school catalogue for the first time listed a laboratory course in pharmacology, taught by Abel's successor, Arthur Cushny. The course was an elective "obtained only by permission," and was aimed at students taking the optional four-year Bachelor of Science in Pharmacy rather than at students in the standard two-year pharmacy program. The lecture course, however, was no longer shown in the pharmacy school catalogue.[71]

A few other pharmacy schools began to introduce more material on the physiological action of drugs into their materia medica courses around the turn of the century, but the most far-reaching effort to teach pharmacology to pharmacy students took place at the University of Nebraska. In 1908, Rufus Lyman, a physician and professor of physiology and pharmacology at the University of Nebraska School of Medicine, accepted an offer to organize a school of pharmacy at Nebraska. Lyman strongly believed that pharmacy education was in need of revitalization through the introduction of more biological science into the curriculum. Hence the new school that he established included pharmacology in its curriculum right from the start, along with zoology, bacteriology, and physiology.

The Nebraska pharmacology course was required in each of the three different pharmacy curricula (two, three, and four years) offered at the university at the time. It consisted of four hours each of lectures and laboratory work for one semester. Nebraska was apparently the first American school of pharmacy to require a course in pharmacology that included both lectures and laboratory work as part of the standard two-year curriculum. Unlike the situation at Michigan, the course was not taught in the medical school, but in the school of pharmacy by Lyman himself.[72]

Lyman's ideas were by no means widely adopted at first, and pharmacology continued to encounter opposition from those who failed to understand why the pharmacist needed to know much about the physiological action of medicines. Critics of the inclusion of significant pharmacological instruction in pharmaceutical education argued that the proper role of the pharmacist was the preparation of medicines, and that he should not encroach upon the physician's domain by placing too much emphasis on the physiological and therapeutic properties of drugs. Some feared that too much knowledge of this sort would tempt pharmacists into prescribing at the drugstore counter.[73]

The efforts of Lyman and others eventually began to bear fruit, however, and by 1920 one survey showed that seventeen of fifty-one pharmacy schools included in the report offered a course in pharmacology. Nine others also claimed to include some pharmacology instruction in another course. A growing interest in the biological assay of drugs, a method based on measuring physiological responses to the administration of drugs (see chapter 5), probably contributed to the growth of pharmacology in pharmacy schools, for it was believed that the pharmacist should have an understanding of such principles. Efforts to base the education of pharmacists more firmly on the underlying pharmaceutical sciences also no doubt assisted the cause of those pressing for more pharmacology in the curriculum.

By the late 1930s, another survey showed that almost all American schools of pharmacy offered some instruction in pharmacology. The quantity and quality of this instruction still varied significantly. For example, less than half of the pharmacy schools offered laboratory work in the subject. In addition, the course was often taught by someone who was not a pharmacologist, and who was responsible for instruction in several different subjects. Nevertheless, pharmacology had gained a strong foothold in schools of pharmacy in the two decades between the First and Second World Wars, even if it had to await the advent of clinical pharmacy to achieve prominence in pharmaceutical education.[74]

The Beginnings of Graduate Education in Pharmacology

While pharmacology was beginning to make inroads into schools of pharmacy during the interwar period, it also continued to expand its role in the nation's medical schools, although some pharmacologists expressed concerns that their field still did not receive the attention that it deserved relative to other subjects in the curriculum (see chapter 6). By the late 1930s, forty-eight of the nation's sixty-six four-year medical schools had independent departments of pharmacology. In the other schools, pharmacology was combined with another department, generally physiology or biochemistry.[75]

As noted earlier, the first generation of American pharmacologists was largely trained as physicians and possessed the M.D. degree, although there were also a few recruits to the field who held Ph.D. degrees in areas such as chemistry. Generally these individuals received whatever specific pharmacological training they obtained by working in the laboratories and assisting in the teaching duties of established pharmacologists. At first this training occurred in Europe, especially in the institute of Schmiedeberg at Strassburg, but later it occurred in the American laboratories of Abel, Cushny, Sollmann, and others.

Pharmacology was dominated by M.D.'s for a longer period than were most preclinical medical sciences. For example, in 1932, a total of 71 percent of medical school faculty teaching pharmacology held an M.D. degree or an M.D. and a Ph.D. degree. The corresponding figure for physiologists was 48 percent. Just about half of the pharmacology group (49 percent) held only the M.D. degree, as compared to a third (34 percent) of the physiologists. Of the forty-eight chairs of independent departments of pharmacology noted in an American Medical Association report published in 1940, forty had medical degrees.[76]

In 1936 Charles Edmunds argued the case for keeping the teaching of pharmacology in the hands of medical graduates:

> There would not seem to be the slightest doubt but that the men who teach pharmacology should possess a medical degree. I am not denying that the training leading to the Ph.D. degree may not be satisfactory for teachers of anatomy, physiology or biochemistry, but pharmacology is so closely interwoven with medicine in its many aspects that a knowledge of disease, such as is gained in a medical course, would seem to be essential.[77]

As discussed earlier, Abel was opposed to establishing a Ph.D. program in pharmacology at Johns Hopkins, and his protégés were M.D.'s or Ph.D.'s who received postdoctoral training in his laboratory. Abel believed that the ideal preparation for a pharmacologist involved training in both medicine and basic sciences such as chemistry. Another leading pharmacologist, Paul Hanzlik of Stanford University, was still firmly opposed to Ph.D. programs in pharmacology in the late 1940s, arguing that the subject was a medical discipline and should remain as such.

In spite of arguments that pharmacology was a basic biological science and was relevant in areas other than medicine, many of its practitioners believed that it was nevertheless tied more closely to the health fields than were some other biomedical sciences. There was, after all, no corresponding pharmacological field to subjects such as plant physiology and plant biochemistry. The absence of a demand for a specialized doctoral program in their subject by many of the leaders in the field did not help the cause of establishing pharmacology as an independent discipline.[78]

In spite of this opposition to graduate degrees in pharmacology, a small number of doctoral programs in the subject did begin to emerge from about the time of the First World War. The history of Ph.D. programs in the biomedical sciences in American medical schools is a subject that has been almost completely ignored by historians, although one author claimed in 1973 that perhaps "the greatest single change in American medical schools over the past few decades has been the growth of Ph.D. training within their walls."[79] Suffice it to say that by the time of the First World War a number of medical schools were offering graduate study leading to advanced degrees in the medical sciences. A 1919 report of a committee of the Association of American Medical Colleges stated that the "common practice" of awarding a Ph.D. for work done in one of the preclinical sciences was well established in, and approved by, medical schools (although admitting that there was controversy over whether the Ph.D. should be granted for research in clinical fields).[80] The American Medical Association's study of medical education in the period 1934–39 reported that fifty-one of the sixty-six four-year medical schools had some relation to the respective graduate schools in their universities, and went on to state:

> In some universities the entire responsibility for the education of graduate students in one or more of the fundamental or clinical medical sciences was assumed by the graduate school; in others this responsibility was vested entirely in the faculty of the school of medicine; in still others administrative responsibility, in whole or in part, was vested in the graduate school, while educational and professional responsibility was vested in the school of medicine, or in a selected group of faculty members who were members of a graduate faculty.[81]

An example of a pioneering graduate program is the one operated by the University of Minnesota School of Medicine in conjunction with the Mayo Foundation. In 1930 the dean of the university's graduate school reported that the program had conferred a total of fifty-three Ph.D. degrees in its fourteen years of existence, thirty-one in basic sciences and twenty-two in clinical subjects. The University of Rochester's School of Medicine has had a doctoral program since its founding in 1925, and was granting between sixteen and twenty-four Ph.D. degrees a year during the 1930s.[82]

At a few schools, it was possible to obtain a Ph.D. degree in pharmacology before 1920. For example, at Cornell University Medical College one could pursue studies leading to a Ph.D. in pharmacology by 1913. Yale University School of Medicine accepted pharmacology as a Ph.D. subject beginning in 1917. At least one student was enrolled in the graduate program with a major in pharmacology at the University of Minnesota by 1917.[83]

It has not been possible to determine when these early programs graduated their first doctoral students. The doctoral program at Cornell Medical College remained a very small one, at least through the 1920s. There were almost never more than half a dozen Ph.D. students enrolled in all fields in the Medical College graduate program, nor more than one Ph.D. granted, in any given year during that period. It is not clear that any of the three students majoring in pharmacology at the University of Minnesota through the 1920–21 academic year actually completed a Ph.D. degree there, although one received his M.S. degree from Minnesota and then went on to earn a Ph.D. in physiology at the University of Chicago.[84]

Several pharmacologists earned doctoral degrees by the early 1920s through pharmacology subunits in other departments, such as physiology, or in joint departments. For example, in 1913 Arthur Tatum earned his doctorate in the Department of Physiology at the University of Chicago, which subsumed pharmacology and physiological chemistry. At the time he received his degree, Tatum was already serving as an instructor in pharmacology and toxicology under Arthur Loevenhart at the University of Wisconsin in Madison, some 150 miles from Chicago. He went on to receive an M.D. degree from Rush Medical College in Chicago in 1914, eventually succeeding Loevenhart at Wisconsin.[85]

In 1917 pharmacology and physiological chemistry at Chicago split off from physiology to form a joint department. Harry Van Dyke, who was later to head the pharmacology departments at Chicago and Columbia as well as at the Squibb Institute for Medical Research, received his Ph.D. from this joint department in 1921. Another prominent pharmacologist, Erwin Nelson, whose career included service in academia, government, and industry, obtained his doctorate from the Department of Physiology and Pharmacology at the University of Missouri in 1920. That pharmacologists still regarded medical credentials as necessary, however, is reflected in the fact that both Van Dyke and Nelson, like Tatum, went on to earn the M.D. degree.[86]

As the 1920s advanced, the number of pharmacology graduate programs increased, albeit at a slow pace. In 1924, for example, the first Ph.D. degrees in pharmacology were awarded at the University of Wisconsin. In 1928 Tulane University granted its first doctoral degree in the field.[87]

It was not until after the Second World War that graduate education in pharmacology began to boom. As late as 1951, one pharmacologist complained that there were still only about a dozen well-organized graduate programs in pharmacology in the United States. Compare this figure to the 132 pharmacology graduate programs in American medical schools listed in a 1988 guide (in addition to 56 more graduate programs in schools of pharmacy and veterinary medicine).[88] By the early 1950s, about half of those teaching pharmacology in medical schools in the United States had Ph.D. degrees, as opposed to approximately one-third with M.D. degrees and one-fifth with both degrees.[89] By 1968 members of the American Society for Pharmacology and Experimental Therapeutics holding a Ph.D. degree outnumbered M.D. members by two to one. Pharmacology was increasingly dominated by those possessing specialized research degrees. Even so, in 1968 the majority of those heading academic pharmacology programs in medical schools still had an M.D. degree or both the M.D. and Ph.D. degrees.[90]

Although American pharmacology first became established as a discipline within academic institutions, and continued to thrive in this setting, pharmacologists were increasingly presented with career options beyond academic research and teaching, as the need for their services in government and industry grew. Indeed, by 1968 somewhat fewer than half of the members of the American Society for Pharmacology and Experimental Therapeutics held positions in university departments of pharmacology.[91]

CHAPTER FIVE

Pharmacologists in Government and Industry

Pharmacology in the Federal Government

Between 1890 and 1910, when experimental pharmacology was replacing materia medica in the curricula of the better American medical schools, the new science was also beginning to find a place in various government and industrial laboratories. Jobs in these environments, and particularly those in industry, were not considered as prestigious within the profession as university appointments, but non-academic laboratories over time came to employ a significant number of pharmacologists. At first, industrial pharmacologists were not even accepted to membership in the national professional society, a situation that was not remedied until the 1940s. This chapter will examine the growth of pharmacology outside of the university setting, beginning with the federal government.

By the time the American Society for Pharmacology and Experimental Therapeutics was created in 1908, its eighteen founding members included five who worked for the federal government.[1] These pharamacologists were based in the two agencies where the science especially flourished during its early years, the Hygienic Laboratory of the Public Health Service (PHS) and the Bureau of Chemistry of the Department of Agriculture. Pharmacology still plays a major role today in the agencies which grew out of these institutions: the National Institutes of Health (NIH), successor to the Hygienic Laboratory, and the Food and Drug Administration (FDA), which was created to assume the regulatory functions of the Bureau of Chemistry. Any consideration of pharmacology within the federal government thus might logically focus largely on these two institutions.

The first appointment of a pharmacologist in a federal agency appears to have been in the Hygienic Laboratory in 1904. The Hygienic Laboratory had been established in Staten Island, New York, by the Marine Hospital Service (later the Public Health Service) in 1887, largely to undertake bacteriological work in connection with public health. In 1891 the laboratory was moved to Washington, D.C. Very little original research was carried out in the first decade or so of the laboratory's existence, but laws passed in 1901 and 1902 reorganized the laboratory and greatly strengthened its research function. As pointed out by Harden and Dupree, it was during the Progressive Era that science became firmly established within the federal government.[2]

One of the changes introduced by the 1902 Act to Increase the Efficiency and Change the Name of the United States Public Health and Marine Hospital Service was to authorize the creation of three new divisions. The existing program was designated the Division of Pathology and Bacteriology, and new Divisions of Chemistry, Pharmacology, and Zoology were created. The fact that pharmacology was one of the divisions established at this time is further evidence of the growing recognition of this relatively new discipline in America.[3] The individual appointed to head the Division of Pharmacology was Abel protégé Reid Hunt (see chapter 4), who began work at the Hygienic Laboratory on 1 March 1904.[4]

The work of the new Division of Pharmacology was divided between research and practical applications of pharmacological knowledge and techniques. The examination of drugs for strength and purity, for example, occupied a significant portion of the staff time in the division. The medical purveyor of the Public Health Service sent samples of drugs to the Pharmacology Division, which tested these drugs against the standards set in the *United States Pharmacopeia* in order to make a recommendation as to whether they should be accepted or rejected. In fiscal year 1905, for example, the division tested 289 drug samples, and found that about one-third of them did not meet acceptable standards.[5]

The division also soon became involved in a major way in public service work with two private professional medical bodies concerned with the quality of the country's drug supply. The problem of the control and standardization of drugs had become an important issue in the United States in the early years of the twentieth century. In 1902, the Biologics Control Act, the earliest piece of Progressive Era health legislation, was passed in an effort to regulate the sale of the recently introduced vaccines and antitoxins. The law was motivated by a 1901 tragedy in which thirteen children in St. Louis died from receiving diphtheria antitoxin contaminated with tetanus. The law directly involved the Hygienic Laboratory in regulatory matters by making the laboratory's Division of Pathology and Bacteriology responsible for annually inspecting the laboratories of the manufacturers of biologics, for testing the preparations for purity, and for determining potency as standard strengths were developed. Licenses were issued to firms that met these standards.[6]

The Biologics Control Act was only the prelude to broader reforms in the area of food and drug control. Rising concern over food and drug adulteration and patent medicine quackery contributed to the movement for a national pure food and drug law, culminating in the passage of the Pure Food and Drugs Act of 1906. Clearly the new science of pharmacology, involving experimental investigations of the actions of drugs and poisons, was relevant to food and drug regulation issues.[7]

Since its founding in 1820, the *United States Pharmacopeia* had attempted to establish standards for drugs, although these standards were not legally enforceable by the federal government until the passage of the 1906 act. The *Pharmacopeia* was not published by a government agency, but by a private body (called "the United States Pharmacopeial Convention" since 1900) consisting of physicians and pharmacists, which was responsible for periodically revising the work. Almost from its very beginning the Division of Pharmacology cooperated with the Pharmacopeial Convention, and with committees of the American Medical Association (AMA) and the American Pharmaceutical Association which were concerned with the *Pharmacopeia*, in efforts to improve drug standards.[8] For example, Hunt and his colleagues undertook experimental work on the standardization of thyroid preparations, and the division published a bulletin in 1905 on changes in the eighth decennial revision of the *Pharmacopeia*.[9]

This cooperation with the *Pharmacopeia* was strongly supported by Milton Rosenau, director of the Hygienic Laboratory, who believed that the Division of Pharmacology was "peculiarly fitted" for work on the physiological standards for drugs and chemicals and that both the division and the *Pharmacopeia* stood to benefit from close relations between them.[10] In his annual report for 1909, the surgeon general of the Public Health Service also argued the case for involvement of the Hygienic Laboratory in pharmacopeial work, largely on the grounds that the 1906 act had made the standards of the *Pharmacopeia* legally enforceable under federal law.[11]

The Division of Pharmacology also became very involved in the work of another body concerned with the quality and safety of drugs, the American Medical Association's Council on Pharmacy and Chemistry. The council had been created in 1905 to investigate the composition and standing of proprietary medicines. The council made recommendations, for example, as to whether or not certain proprietary medicines deserved the patronage of physicians and pharmacists, and whether or not the AMA's journal should accept advertising for these products. Beginning in 1907, the council issued *New and Nonofficial Remedies,* an annual publication which provided physicians and pharmacists with information on drug products not included in the *United States Pharmacopeia* or the *National Formulary.*[12]

From the establishment of the council in early 1905, Martin Wilbert, a pharmacist in the Hygienic Laboratory's Division of Pharmacology, was a member. A year later, Reid Hunt joined Wilbert as a member of the council, and remained one for thirty years. The Division of Pharmacology undertook various investigations for the council, examining the composition, activity, or toxicity of specific drug products.[13]

The Division of Pharmacology was also sometimes called upon to assist other government agencies. For example, division staff cooperated on a number of occasions with the Bureau of Chemistry of the Department of Agriculture in connection with the evaluation of drugs or chemicals, since the bureau was responsible for the enforcement of the 1906 Pure Food and Drugs Act (see below). Other agencies assisted by the division included the army (testing the physiological activity of certain adrenal gland preparations), the Interior Department (examining the radioactivity of the waters of Hot Springs, Arkansas), and the Post Office Department (regarding exclusion from the mails of certain fraudulent medicines).[14]

In addition to these activities, which were more or less directly related to public health and the enforcement of drug standards, the division also engaged in a significant amount of basic research in pharmacology. At first the practical work of the division occupied almost all of Hunt's attention. The report of the division for 1905, for example, noted that there had been little time during the year for systematic research work.[15] In March of that year, Director Rosenau complained to the surgeon general: "Dr. Hunt has a special genius for original research in physiological chemistry and has many problems in mind which offer results of the greatest value if he could be relieved of most of the routine work of examining drugs and chemicals."[16]

Later reports of the division indicate that research soon became one of its important functions. Hunt and his colleagues explored such subjects as the physiology and pharmacology of thyroid preparations and the pharmacology of alcohol.[17] The most significant research to come out of the division in its early years was Hunt's study with Taveau on the physiological action of choline derivatives in the period 1906–11. In the course of this work, they observed the remarkable activity of acetylcholine, reporting that this substance was one hundred thousand times more potent itself than choline in lowering the blood pressure.[18] It was not until the 1920s, however, that the role of acetylcholine in the chemical transmission of nervous impulses was established through the work of Otto Loewi in Austria and Henry Dale in England.

On the basis of these many activities, especially those concerned with public health, Hunt argued successfully for expansion of the staff of the division. Arrangements were also made for academic scientists to spend time working in the division on a temporary basis. For example, Cornell University pharmacologist Robert Hatcher spent the summer of 1909 working in the Hygienic Laboratory on the determination of some of the physical constants of pharmacopeial substances, and pharmacologist C. W. Edmunds of the University of Michigan spent the summer of 1910 there working on methods for the standardization of ergot. Such arrangements helped to forge closer ties between the division and university centers of pharmacological research.[19]

An examination of the division's report for 1910 provides at least a qualitative breakdown of the work of the division in one typical year under Hunt's leadership. Significant attention was devoted to a study of methods to improve the standardization of digitalis, epinephrine, and thyroid extract, since commercial preparations of all of these drugs were found to vary greatly in their strength. An investigation of the possible injurious effects of bleached flour on man was carried out and the results incorporated into a bulletin published by the Hygienic Laboratory. Other research work in the division involved the physiology and pharmacology of the thyroid gland, anaphylaxis, the pharmacology of choline and similar compounds, corn meal and corn oil as foodstuffs (in connection with the disease pellagra), and the toxicity of mixtures containing acetanilide and caffeine or para-amidophenol. Reports on some of these studies were delivered at professional meetings and published in scientific journals. The division also carried out routine examinations of some 120 drugs, largely those purchased by the purveyor for use in the marine hospitals. In addition, members of the division served on various committees and boards of professional associations such as the American Medical Association and the American Pharmaceutical Association. Hunt attended several professional meetings during the year, including a national conference on pellagra, the Twelfth International Congress on Alcoholism in London, and the Sixteenth International Medical Congress in Budapest.[20]

In 1913 Reid Hunt left the Hygienic Laboratory to become professor of pharmacology at Harvard University (see chapter 4). His successor was another protégé of John Abel, Carl Voegtlin, who like Hunt, was widely respected in his field. While at the Hygienic Laboratory, Voegtlin carried out important research on the chemotherapy of organic arsenic compounds. It was also during Voegtlin's tenure that the Division of Pharmacology became responsible for the chemical and pharmacological testing of preparations of the arsenical drug Salvarsan (given the generic name "arsphenamine" in the United States). In 1910 Salvarsan had been introduced in Germany by Paul Ehrlich as a treatment for syphilis and for certain infections caused by the microorganisms known as trypanosomes, and had quickly become an important chemotherapeutic agent. When the United States entered World War I, German patent rights were abrogated and approved American manufacturers were allowed to produce arsphenamine. Because of the difficulty in obtaining uniform preparations of the drug, manufacturers were required to test each lot for toxicity and arsenic content. Samples also had to be submitted to the Hygienic Laboratory for possible testing by this agency.[21]

In 1930 the Hygienic Laboratory became the National Institute of Health and significantly expanded its activities. The Division of Pharmacology remained a branch of the new National Institute of Health, still under the leadership of Voegtlin. When the National Cancer Institute was established in 1937, Voegtlin was selected as its first director, but he continued to serve as chief of the Division of Pharmacology until 1940.[22] As the number of institutes devoted to different disease conditions increased, and the agency became the National Institutes of Health, pharmacology was no longer centered in one specific division. Today pharmacologists may be employed in any one of the NIH institutes in a variety of laboratory settings.

Since the Public Health Service began to concern itself with the health of workers beginning around 1910, one might expect that pharmacologists would have been employed within the PHS by the 1920s to study industrial toxicology, but this was not the case. Although the PHS did developed an interest in occupational toxicology, this interest was not translated into significant efforts in laboratory toxicology or pharmacology during the time period emphasized in this book. The agency's Office of Industrial Hygiene and Sanitation, organized in 1919, concentrated on field studies and statistical reports, rather than on laboratory studies of the toxicology of industrial substances. The Bureau of Mines (in the Department of the Interior until 1925, when it was transferred to the Department of Commerce) did carry out laboratory investigations related to occupational toxicology, often in collaboration with the PHS, but even these studies were more pathological and chemical than pharmacological in nature, and were directed by surgeon Royd R. Sayers. Professional pharmacologists played only a peripheral role in the emerging field of industrial toxicology. Although a handful of pharmacologists (including government scientists E. W. Schwartze of the United States Department of Agriculture's Bureau of Chemistry and Carl Voegtlin of the Public Health Services' Hygienic Laboratory) were among the eighty-eight representatives of government, industrial, and academic institutions at a 1925 conference on the health hazards of tetraethyl lead gasoline, organized by the PHS surgeon general, none of them was a formal speaker on the program.[23]

The federal agency other than the Hygienic Laboratory where the science of pharmacology began to make its impact felt at an early date was the Bureau of Chemistry of the Department of Agriculture. Physician and chemist Harvey Wiley, who had served as chief of the Bureau from 1883, was the major figure responsible for the passage of the 1906 Pure Food and Drugs Act. The enforcement of the provisions of the act had been placed in the hands of Wiley's Bureau of Chemistry, and he recognized early the need for a pharmacologist to help in carrying out these regulatory responsibilities.

In March 1908, pharmaceutical chemist Lyman Kebler, chief of the Bureau of Chemistry's Division of Drugs, wrote to John Abel seeking his advice on the employment of a pharmacologist: "We are desirous of securing some one qualified in pharmacology and would ask if you are acquainted with any one whom you would care to recommend for our work. It is chiefly in connection with the enforcement of the Food and Drugs Act."[24]

Abel recommended a former associate of his, A. C. Crawford, who was then employed by the Department of Agriculture's Bureau of

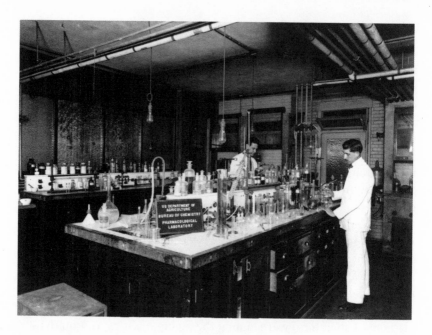

Pharmacological laboratory at the Bureau of Chemistry, United States Department of Agriculture, about the time of World War I.

Courtesy of the History Office, United States Food and Drug Administration.

Plant Industry.[25] Either Kebler did not accept this advice or Crawford did not accept the job, for in June of that year William Salant was appointed to head the newly created pharmacological laboratory in the bureau's Division of Drugs.[26] Salant received an M.D. from the College of Physicians and Surgeons at Columbia University and then spent the next several years as an assistant in physiology or physiological chemistry at the Cornell and Columbia medical schools, while also carrying out research under grants from the Rockefeller Institute for Medical Research. He was serving as an adjunct professor at the University of Alabama when he was hired by the Bureau of Chemistry.[27]

The research that was carried out at first in the bureau's pharmacological laboratory seems to have largely grown out of regulatory concerns. For example, among the subjects extensively studied in the early years of the laboratory were the physiological effects of extracts of bleached and unbleached flour and the pharmacology and toxicology of caffeine.[28] Both of these studies were directly related to court cases which involved the bureau. Wiley was opposed to the practice of bleaching flour with nitrogen peroxide, as he felt it involved the use of an objectionable substance for the unethical purpose of concealing an inferior product. The studies of the pharmacological laboratory on flour were obviously designed to determine whether the bleached flour might have undesirable physiological effects. Wiley also objected to the addition of caffeine to Coca-Cola, arguing that it was a poisonous ingredient. Again, the research in the pharmacological laboratory on the pharmacology and toxicology of caffeine was carried out in support of Wiley's regulatory efforts.[29] In discussing the work of the laboratory, the 1911 report of the bureau clearly stated that "much of the information acquired on the physiological effect of various drugs and chemicals was used in connection with the enforcement of the food and drugs act and the preparation of expert testimony along these lines."[30] Bureau pharmacologists also sometimes found themselves on the witness stand describing their toxicological experiments in some of the cases prosecuted by the bureau.[31]

Although much of the research of the pharmacological laboratory was motivated by practical concerns, the results were sometimes of broader scientific interest, and Salant and his colleagues (like Hunt and his co-workers) reported on some of their work at professional meetings and in the scientific literature.[32] On the whole, however, the Bureau of Chemistry's pharmacological laboratory was less oriented toward basic research than the Hygienic Laboratory's Division of Pharmacology, and neither Salant nor his immediate successors ever achieved the status in the field enjoyed by Hunt and Voegtlin, both of whom eventually served as presidents of the American Society for Pharmacology and Experimental Therapeutics. In discussing the Bureau of Chemistry, it should be noted that a biochemist-pharmacologist, Carl Alsberg, succeeded Wiley as chief of the bureau in 1912. During Alsberg's tenure, which lasted until 1921, the bureau became more research oriented.[33]

In addition to the efforts of its own pharmacologists, by the 1920s the Bureau of Chemistry was also making significant use of the services of outside pharmacologists for advice and expert testimony. Wisconsin pharmacologist Arthur Loevenhart, for example, served as an expert witness for the Bureau of Chemistry on several trials involving the toxicity of lead arsenate pesticide residues on fruit. Reid Hunt headed a committee appointed by the bureau at the end of 1926 to provide "the best available opinion upon the limits of lead and arsenic which shall be tolerated in human foods." The committee also included pharmacologists Loevenhart and Carl Voegtlin, as well as former bureau chief Carl Alsberg.[34]

In 1927 the Food, Drug, and Insecticide Administration was created within the Department of Agriculture, and the regulatory responsibilities for the food and drug law were transferred from the Bureau of Chemistry to this new agency. In 1930 the agency was renamed the Food and Drug Administration.[35] The FDA remained a part of the Department of Agriculture until 1940, when it was transferred to the new Federal Security Agency (which was replaced by the Department of Health, Education, and Welfare in 1953).

Pharmacology was given a major boost within the FDA when a separate Division of Pharmacology was established in 1935. The annual report of the agency for that year noted that "the importance of fundamental researches in pharmacology to furnish a groundwork for food-and-drug law enforcement led to the establishment during the year of the Pharmacological Division." The report singled out two special areas of interest of the new division. One of these areas was the biological assay of various medicinal products on the market, such as glandular preparations. In addition to carrying out FDA's regulatory function of sampling and testing interstate shipment of these products, the division was also expected to develop new methods for identifying and determining the strength and purity of medicaments. A second area emphasized in the report was the study of the toxicity (especially the chronic effects) of substances used as food additives or which occurred as impurities in foods (e.g., insecticide residues).[36]

Erwin Nelson, who was at the time associate professor of pharmacology at the University of Michigan, was persuaded to take a two-year leave of absence from his academic post to launch the new division. One of the early appointees to the staff of the division recalled that at first there was "a preponderance of biochemists who then changed sails and became pharmacologists." Chemical expertise may have been given special attention at this time because the division's initial focus was heavily on toxicology. The controversy over the toxic effects of lead arsenate insecticide spray residues on fruit, for example, was an important factor in the establishment of the Division of Pharmacology.[37]

The 1936 report of the division noted that new laboratories and animal quarters for pharmacological investigation had been equipped, and that a long-term research project on the chronic toxicity of lead and arsenic was underway. A large colony of experimental animals was allotted to the division for the study of various glandular products. During the year the division carried out biological assays on 399 drugs and drug preparations.[38]

The passage of the 1938 Food, Drug, and Cosmetic Act significantly expanded the scope of the FDA's power and increased its need for scientific staff, including pharmacologists. For example, the act required manufacturers to test a new drug for safety and to obtain FDA clearance before marketing the product. The law also brought cosmetics under the control of the FDA for the first time. In 1939, an interest in the safety of cosmetics led the FDA to hire pharmacologist John Draize, a Wisconsin Ph.D. who specialized in dermal toxicity. Working at the FDA, in 1944 Draize developed the well-known and now controversial test for eye toxicity that bears his name. Pharmacology has continued to expand at the Food and Drug Administration over the past few decades, and the agency remains today as a significant employer of professional pharmacologists within the federal government.[39]

In addition to the efforts in the Bureau of Chemistry and later in the FDA, some pharmacological work was also carried out in two other divisions of the Department of Agriculture as early as the first decade of the twentieth century. The pharmacological research in the Bureau of Plant Industry centered on poisonous plants, an interest of the bureau since 1894. About 1902, even before the bureau had hired a pharmacologist, a botanist on its staff was collaborating with academic pharmacologists Reid Hunt (then at Johns Hopkins) and Torald Sollmann (at Western Reserve) on studies of poisonous plants. Albert C. Crawford, mentioned above, was the first pharmacologist employed by the Bureau of Plant Industry. He appears to have been appointed in the summer of 1904 or not long afterward. Crawford received a medical degree from the College of Physicians and Surgeons of Baltimore before becoming an assistant in Abel's laboratory. He remained in the Bureau of Plant Industry until 1908, when he moved to the Department of Agriculture's Bureau of Animal Industry, apparently as their first pharmacologist. There he continued his investigations on the pharmacology of poisonous plants. He was replaced in the Bureau of Plant Industry by Carl Alsberg.[40]

Pharmacology thus became established in federal agencies such as the Hygienic Laboratory and the Bureau of Chemistry in the first decade of the twentieth century. The new science found its way into these agencies largely as a result of public health concerns, especially about the nation's food and drug supply, but also at least in part as a result of increasing interest in scientific research in federal laboratories. Regulatory legislation enacted during the Progressive Era helped to promote the expansion of scientific staffs in federal agencies and their increasing involvement in research. The science of pharmacology was included in this broader trend.[41]

Before leaving the subject of the federal government, at least brief mention must be made of the beginnings of modern pharmacology in the military, which occurred in the Chemical Warfare Service during World War I. When the United States entered the war in 1917, there was no American military or government agency responsible for dealing with gas warfare. The Bureau of Mines, which had been established in 1908, was the only agency that had significant relevant experience due to its concern with explosive and poisonous gases in mines, self-contained breathing apparatus, and the treatment of those exposed to noxious gases. The bureau offered its services to the War Department, which gladly accepted the offer.

In addition to the creation of a central laboratory at the American University in Washington, D.C., various branch laboratories of the Bureau of Mines were established at universities and other institutions around the country to investigate chemical warfare. Yandell Henderson, professor of physiology at Yale University, was given the responsibility of organizing the research on the medical problems associated with gas warfare. By June 1918, President Wilson had authorized the creation of the Chemical Warfare Service as a branch of the United States Army, and the military assumed the role of chief coordinator and director of the chemical warfare work.

Obviously, expertise in pharmacology and toxicology was of value in gas warfare research, and not surprisingly pharmacologists became involved in the work of the Chemical Warfare Service. Most prominent among these were Arthur Loevenhart of Wisconsin and E. K. Marshall, Jr., of Johns Hopkins, both protégés of Abel. Loevenhart headed the pharmacological and toxicological section that dealt with problems of offense—that is, the section's functions were to develop economical methods of making the gases used by the Germans and to develop more effective gases. Marshall headed the pharmacological unit concerned with problems of defense—that is, the unit's functions were to study the mode of action and effects of the gases in use and the general susceptibility of men to poisoning.

As an example of how Loevenhart's offense unit (which consisted of about 150 workers) operated, a potentially toxic compound would be synthesized and then tested on a small scale for toxicity on laboratory animals. Attention was also devoted to methods of dispersing the compound. If the compound seemed promising, larger amounts were produced for field studies with animals, culminating in a large-scale test simulating battle conditions.[42]

World War I stimulated American research in chemistry and other disciplines through efforts such as the Chemical Warfare Service. In addition, American firms cut off from their usual German supply of chemicals and pharmaceuticals were forced to become more actively involved in the production of synthetic chemicals. After the United States entered the conflict in 1917, German patents were seized and made available to American manufacturers under license. The American pharmaceutical and chemical industries were given a significant boost by the war.[43]

Pharmacologists in Industry

The emergence of the industrial research laboratory dates back to the late nineteenth century, with its roots in the German coal-tar dye industry. As dye firms such as Friedrich Bayer and Company expanded into the pharmaceutical market, their research activities began to encompass the development and testing of new chemical substances for their therapeutic potential. By the beginning of the twentieth century, pharmaceutical research was well established in German industrial firms, which often had close ties to the universities.[44]

With few exceptions, research in American industrial firms remained unorganized and largely nonexistent until the twentieth century. Many of the major American pharmaceutical companies did, however, establish laboratories in the late nineteenth century. The goal of these laboratories was generally not research aimed at the development of new products or innovation in general, but rather the standardization of the quantity and quality of ingredients and the potency of existing products. Nevertheless, for the first time these firms began to hire chemists, pharmacists, and physicians for analytical laboratory work. These analytical laboratories also sometimes became involved in aspects of the control of manufacturing processes.

Science thus began to enter the American pharmaceutical industry, even if, as Jonathan Liebenau claims, it was at first more of a veneer than a driving force. Companies that could promise to deliver standardized preparations had an edge in winning the confidence of the public and the health professions. Thus, in 1881 Parke, Davis and Company hired physician Albert B. Lyons to establish a systematic program of assaying and standardizing alkaloidal drugs and fluid extracts. In the mid-1880s, Eli Lilly and Company established a Scientific Department, largely an analytical laboratory at first, with graduate pharmacists Josiah K. Lilly and Ernest G. Eberhardt serving as chemists. Another pharmacy school graduate, Lyman F. Kebler, was appointed chief chemist and asked to organize an analytical laboratory at Smith, Kline and Company.[45]

At first these efforts to standardize drugs were voluntary, but with the passage of the Pure Food and Drugs Act of 1906 the standards established for medicaments in the *Pharmacopeia of the United States* and the *National Formulary* acquired the force of law. Coupled with the earlier 1902 act regulating the production and sale of biologicals, this meant that the assaying and standardization of drugs was no longer a luxury, but the cost of doing business. Laboratories and scientific workers thus became an integral part of ethical pharmaceutical firms, eventually leading to the development of research programs.[46]

Initially, standardization was carried out by chemical means. It soon became apparent, however, that the application of chemical procedures was inadequate for determining the active principle in a number of drugs. For example, by the beginning of the twentieth century, some twenty substances had been isolated from ergot, and even these were eventually shown to be mixtures. Although there were chemical methods available for estimating the alkaloid content of ergot extracts, no reliable relationship could be established between the determined amount of alkaloids and the strength of the physiological action on the uterus. Similar problems were encountered with other drugs such as digitalis. The problem became even more acute when biological agents such as glandular extracts and antitoxins, whose chemical nature was at first completely unknown, came into therapeutic use toward the end of the nineteenth century.

Some investigators began to use physiological methods to estimate the strength of drug preparations in the late nineteenth century. For example, Albert Frankel in Berlin determined the relative strength of the various digitalis preparations in the German pharmacopeia by recording the rise in blood pressure produced in dogs. On the whole, however, as Peter Stechl has shown in a study of the early history of biological standardization, pharmacologists of the period showed relatively little interest in developing quantitative physiological methods for standardizing drug preparations. Their focus was on the efforts to isolate and study the action of the active chemical principles of crude drugs. At the dawn of experimental pharmacology as a science, Magendie had stressed the importance of isolating active ingredients, and had based his own formulary on such pure principles (see chapter 1). Buchheim also emphasized that the isolation of the active principles was the only means by which uniformity of dosage could be obtained. The successful isolation of a large number of active principles in the nineteenth century no doubt encouraged the belief that chemically pure active ingredients would be obtained from at least most crude drugs in the relatively near future.

Manufacturers of drugs, or at least those concerned with producing standardized products, had more reason to be interested in the potential usefulness of physiological testing. Some early efforts in this direction were made by physician and drug manufacturer Edward R. Squibb, who, in the 1880s, used the ability of belladonna to dilate the pupil of the eye to determine the potency of samples of the crude drug. He defined as a drug of standard strength one that produced a distinct effect on the eye (human or cat) at a dilution of 1:500, but no effect or a scarcely perceptible one at a dilution of 1:600. Although this and other methods used by Squibb produced results that were extremely approximate and variable, they helped to establish the principles and goals of biological standardization.[47]

Just as chemical science entered the pharmaceutical industry in large part because of concerns about drug assay and standardization, pharmacology also seems to have made its way into the industry at first because of the need for standardization, particularly in connection with biological or physiological assay. As previously noted, E. R. Squibb himself began using pharmacological procedures to estimate drug potency in the 1880s. The first individual employed by an American pharmaceutical company whom we can clearly identify as a pharmacologist, however, is Elijah M. Houghton of Parke, Davis and Company.

Houghton was hired by the firm in 1895 in connection with their efforts to produce diphtheria antitoxin. Parke-Davis's interest in this project began when General Manager George Davis read a newspaper account of papers presented by Emil von Behring and by Emile Roux at the International Congress of Hygiene in Budapest in the fall of 1894 on the success of serum therapy for diphtheria using von Behring's antitoxin. Through the efforts of Paul Ehrlich in Germany, a biological standardization procedure had been developed for the antitoxin. According to Peter Stechl, Ehrlich's work in this connection came to serve as a model for biological standardization.[48]

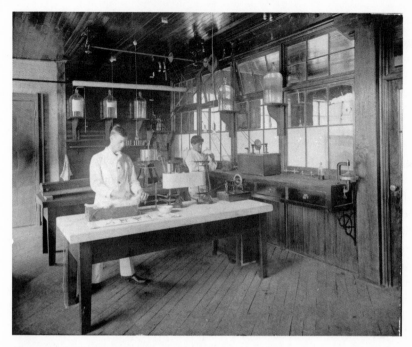

Pharmacological laboratory at Parke, Davis and Company, Detroit, about 1900.

Courtesy of the American Institute of the History of Pharmacy and the F. B. Power Pharmaceutical Library, University of Wisconsin–Madison.

Davis contacted the University of Michigan, where faculty members Frederick Novy and Victor Vaughan (see chapter 2) had just returned from the international congress with information on the antitoxin. Davis was apparently referred to one of Vaughan's associates, Charles T. McClintock, who held both M.D. and Ph.D. degrees. McClintock agreed to assist Parke-Davis in producing the antitoxin. McClintock did not want to leave Ann Arbor, however, because of the research that he was carrying out with Vaughan. Arrangements were therefore made for him to produce the antitoxin in Ann Arbor, and to treat several horses in Detroit.

It soon became apparent, however, that someone in Detroit should be working on the project. McClintock had discussed his antitoxin work from its early stages with Houghton, a colleague at Michigan, and the question arose as to whether Houghton would be willing to go to Detroit to work for Parke-Davis. Houghton had received his M.D. from Michigan in 1894, and was serving as an assistant in pharmacology to Cushny at the time. He was well qualified for the task because he had just begun experiments in the summer or fall of 1894 on biological methods for standardizing digitalis, apparently at the suggestion of Cushny. His interest in standardization may have played a role in his willingness to accept the position at Parke-Davis, which he did after consulting with Cushny and others. Houghton began work in Detroit early in 1895. McClintock meanwhile continued to serve as a consultant on the project until 1896, when he joined the staff of Parke-Davis as director of research. At about that same time, Houghton was given the title of assistant director of research.

Soon after Houghton began work in Detroit, the company was producing its first relatively potent diphtheria antitoxin. Once the production of the antitoxin was underway, McClintock and Houghton were apparently allowed to devote a significant amount of their time to research, making Parke-Davis one of the pioneers of industrial research among American pharmaceutical firms. In 1902 a separate building was constructed for Parke-Davis's research laboratories, one of the first built exclusively for research in any American industry.[49]

Houghton went on to become one of the pioneers in the development of biological standardization techniques, working in the laboratories of Parke-Davis. His research continued to be tied closely to practical concerns of drug standardization. In 1897 the company introduced the first of the plant drugs physiologically standardized by Houghton's work. They included extracts of ergot, cannabis, strophanthus, and digitalis. The firm was pleased to be able to emphasize in its advertisements that physiological testing insured that pharmacists would be dispensing a "reliable fluid extract" of these drugs.[50]

Another physician interested in pharmacology and materia medica, Francis E. Stewart (see below), had tried to interest Parke-Davis in setting up a pharmacological laboratory a decade before the company hired Houghton. At the time, in 1884, Stewart was working as an assistant in the laboratory of Horatio Wood in Philadelphia (see chapter 1). Stewart was also working under contract to Parke-Davis, serving as a special "traveling representative" whose main function seemed to be to promote the company among the medical profession in Philadelphia. Stewart envisioned himself as running the proposed laboratory, but he could not convince George Davis to commit the funds to such a project. He was also unsuccessful in convincing the firm to establish a pharmacological society whose main purpose would be to advance the interests of the industry. It is not surprising that Stewart failed in these efforts at a time when the field of pharmacology had not even seriously begun to establish itself in the United States.[51]

The H. K. Mulford Company in Philadelphia began production of the diphtheria antitoxin at about the same time as Parke-Davis did. Mulford was also one of the early American leaders in industrial research and in ties with the academic scientific community. At first, however, the firm does not appear to have employed anyone who could be called a pharmacologist, although admittedly the subject was just emerging as a distinct discipline in the United States at the time. Antitoxin production at Mulford was supervised by Joseph McFarland, a physician and bacteriologist. McFarland also carried out research aimed at developing antivenoms for snake bites. His work for the company was on a part-time basis, and he continued to teach pathology and bacteriology in Philadelphia medical schools as well as to maintain a small private medical practice. Mulford did, however, secure the services of a bona fide pharmacologist, Torald Sollmann of Western Reserve University, as a consultant at the turn of the century.[52]

By 1909 Mulford was standardizing a significant number of preparations, including botanical drugs as well as biologicals, by physiological assay. In 1910 the company hired pharmacist and pharmaceutical chemist Paul Stewart Pittenger to serve as director of pharmacodynamic research. Although not trained as a pharmacologist, Pittenger developed a special interest in physiological assay and made significant contributions to the field, including the preparation of two textbooks on the subject. In 1911 Pittenger was appointed as special lecturer in pharmacodynamics and physiological standardization of drugs at the Medico-Chirurgical College and at the Philadelphia College of Pharmacy. He thus evolved into a pharmacologist of sorts.[53]

In 1906 Mulford had already hired another self-trained pharmacologist, Francis E. Stewart, as director of its scientific department. Stewart had obtained a pharmacy degree from the Philadelphia College of Pharmacy in 1879 and a medical degree from Jefferson Medical College in 1879. He had practiced medicine in Philadelphia and New York, and also had worked under contract to Parke-Davis before joining the staff of Mulford.[54]

Other pharmaceutical companies also became involved in physiological standardization, although this did not guarantee the firm would employ individuals who identified professionally with pharmacology. As Peter Stechl has noted, pharmacologists were scarce and expensive for carrying out the testing once it had been made routine, and the task was therefore often just added to the work of chemists or others on the staff who could be trained to carry it out. In 1910 pharmacologist H. C. Wood, Jr., complained that biological standardization in American pharmaceutical firms was often carried out by individuals who did not have the necessary qualifications for the work. He recognized, however, that pharmacologists frequently failed to recognize the importance of biological standardization for medicine and left it to the manufacturers, whom Wood felt often saw the procedure largely in terms of its value in advertising. He urged companies to hire trained pharmacologists for this work, and to make the job more appealing to such individuals by giving them scientific freedom.[55]

Research in American industry in general greatly expanded after the First World War, increasing the employment opportunities for pharmacologists and other scientists. One historian has called the 1920s "the seedtime of American industrial laboratories."[56] Such laboratories existed before the war, but the 1920s and 1930s saw a significant growth in the number and size of industrial research laboratories, including those in the pharmaceutical industry. There were qualitative as well as quantitative changes in this research activity. Research in the pharmaceutical industry was upgraded through improved facilities and better-qualified personnel, and greater attention was paid to research of a more fundamental nature. Many scientists who joined the staffs of pharmaceutical firms in the period between the two world wars rose to prominence within their respective disciplines, such as Ernest Henry Volwiler (Abbott Laboratories), G. H. A. Clowes (Eli Lilly), Oliver Kamm (Parke-Davis), and Max Tishler (Merck). Cooperative research with academic scientists was also greatly expanded.[57]

Two examples of how these developments affected industrial pharmacology may be seen at Eli Lilly and at Merck. A Scientific Department had been established at Lilly in the mid-1880s, but there is no evidence to suggest that research was an important function of the unit in its early years. Not surprisingly, the main function of the division initially seems to have been standardization and quality control. Records in the Lilly Archives, for example, document the work on physiological testing of fluid extracts of digitalis, ergot, and other substances carried out in the early years of the twentieth century. In 1911 a separate building was constructed for control and research work, and research activity and the publication of scientific papers on the part of Lilly staff appear to have increased. The new building did contain a pharmacological laboratory.[58]

The first issue of the *Lilly Scientific Bulletin*, published in April 1912, lists two "pharmacologists" on the staff of the Department of Experimental Medicine of the Scientific Department, Charles R. Eckler and W. F. Baker. Eckler was trained as a pharmacist, however, and seems to have had more expertise in chemistry and pharmacognosy than in experimental pharmacology. In fact, in 1920 he was transferred to a chemical research unit at Lilly with the notation on his personal record: "To place in correct Dept." On the other hand, he did carry out pharmacological studies, and he published papers on pharmacological methods for the study and testing of certain drugs. It has not been possible to determine Baker's background, but research records at Lilly indicate that he was performing experiments to determine the relative toxicity of several heart tonics on frogs in 1912.[59]

A number of pharmacological papers were published from the Lilly laboratories in the period before 1920. At least some of these papers met the research standards of the pharmacological profession, as evidenced by the series of studies on the ipecac alkaloids and synthetic derivatives published in the prestigious *Journal of Pharmacology and Experimental Therapeutics* in 1917. The authors were Arthur L. Walters, Edward W. Koch, Eckler, and Baker. Walters, a Johns Hopkins medical graduate, was director of the Division of Experimental Medicine. Koch, who was listed as a pharmacologist on the Lilly staff, had received his medical degree from Rush Medical College in 1911. He spent several years as an assistant and instructor in physiology and pharmacology at Indiana University before being hired by Lilly in 1915.[60]

Research at Lilly, and especially attention to more fundamental research, received a significant boost when G. H. A. Clowes was appointed as a biochemist in 1919 and became director of research the following year. Clowes had strong ties to the academic scientific community and encouraged cooperation between Lilly and university scientists. Clowes and his colleagues, for example, collaborated with scientists at the University of Toronto in the production of insulin, and with scientists at the University of Rochester and Harvard University in the production of liver extracts.[61]

As part of his agreement with Lilly, Clowes was able to spend his summers at the Marine Biological Laboratory in Woods Hole, Massachusetts, pursuing his research interests on subjects such as cancer and cellular respiration. When the Hygienic Laboratory tried to recruit Clowes to be chief of its Division of Pharmacology early in his tenure at Lilly, he turned down the offer because he believed that he had an ideal position for someone primarily concerned with research.

> Eli Lilly and Company have treated me with the greatest generosity. They have created a purely research position for me, in which, for the first time in my life, I am free to devote my attention to those fundamental problems on the border line field of physics, chemistry, biology and medicine, in which, as you doubtless know, I am interested. They have provided me with ample laboratory facilities and assistants and have arranged to let me carry on the biological side of the work at Woods Hole during the summer months.[62]

In spite of the upgrading of research activities under Clowes beginning around 1920, it was not until the end of the decade that Lilly achieved prominence in pharmacological research with the hiring of Ko Kuei Chen. A native of China, Chen had come to the United States for his education, obtaining his B.S. in pharmacy and his Ph.D. in physiology from the University of Wisconsin. After obtaining the latter degree in 1923, he returned to his native country to teach at the Peking Union Medical College. Chen began to concentrate his research efforts on the investigation of traditional Chinese drugs, one of which was Ma Huang (*Ephedra sinica*), which caused a pronounced rise in blood pressure. Chen was able to isolate from the plant the alkaloid that was responsible for the pharmacological activity. He believed that he had discovered a new compound, although he later found that the substance had been isolated in pure form in 1887 by W. Nagayoshi Nagai and named ephedrine. It was Chen and his colleague Carl Schmidt who worked out the pharmacological action and preliminary clinical applications of ephedrine, which soon came into widespread use for bronchial asthma, hay fever, and certain other allergies; ephedrine also played a useful role as an adjunct in spinal and general anesthesia.

With an important discovery already to his credit, Chen left Peking Union in 1925 to return to the United States, this time to Johns Hopkins University, where he obtained his M.D. in 1927. He also worked as an associate in John Abel's laboratory beginning in that same year. Eli Lilly and Company was familiar with Chen's work, since they had begun marketing ephedrine in 1926 and had consulted with Chen about it. The success of ephedrine had aroused the interest of the company's president, J. K. Lilly, in the potential of Chinese materia medica and in the possibility of employing a pharmacologist knowledgeable about the subject. In 1929 Chen was appointed director of pharmacological research at Lilly, a position that he held until his retirement in 1963.

The appointment of Chen placed pharmacological research on a much more organized and substantive footing at Lilly. His scientific contributions included research on the treatment of cyanide poisoning, on cardiac glycosides and toad poisons, on analgesic drugs, on Chinese herbs, and on genetic pharmacology. He went on to become the first industrial scientist to serve as president of the American Society for Pharmacology and Experimental Therapeutics (1952). Chen possessed the necessary credentials and demonstrated the kind of research productivity that made it difficult for his academic colleagues to dismiss him as a "hack" pharmacologist employed by industry to carry out routine assay work.[63]

A similar development occurred at Merck in the early 1930s with the appointment of Hans Molitor. Although Merck and Company had established a research laboratory in the United States as early as 1916, when it was still a branch of the German firm, its early efforts were largely devoted to developing and improving production processes for drugs and other chemicals. The company decided to greatly expand its research activities in 1930, and hired Princeton chemist Randolph Major as director of pure research.[64] At the same time, the firm decided to establish a pharmacological laboratory to evaluate products produced by the expanded chemical research group and also to undertake fundamental research. Merck approached A. Newton Richards of the University of Pennsylvania (chapter 4) in the summer of 1930, asking him to serve as a consultant to the company in their pharmacological efforts. Richards accepted, beginning his consultantship in 1931.[65]

One of Richards's first tasks was to help the firm organize and staff a pharmacology laboratory. The laboratory was to be responsible for a significant amount of routine testing, while also undertaking fundamental pharmacological research. Richards began contacting colleagues both at home and abroad about suitable candidates to head the laboratory. One of those scientists whom he contacted, E. P. Pick, professor of pharmacology at Vienna, suggested Hans Molitor of his own pharmacological institute. Richards had met Molitor in 1927 and was impressed with him, so he urged Merck to recruit him. In 1933 Molitor joined the staff of Merck as director of the Merck Institute for Therapeutic Research, the company's new pharmacological laboratory.[66]

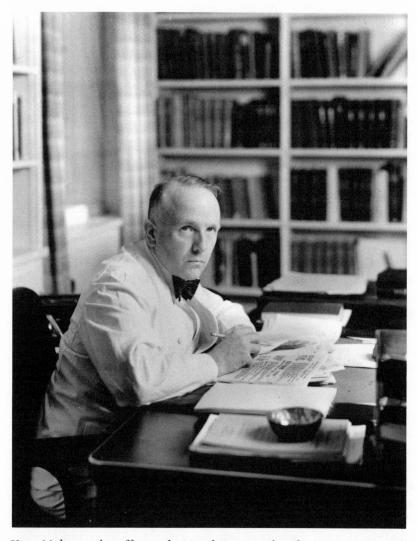

Hans Molitor in his office at the Merck Institute for Therapeutic Research, about 1940.

Courtesy of Merck & Co., Inc., Rahway, N.J.

The pharmacology laboratory was established as a separate non-profit entity at the request of the New Jersey Department of Health in order to comply with a state law for the prevention of cruelty to animals. The law required that animal experiments could only be performed under the authority of the Department of Health, which was granted the power to authorize such experiments at appropriate institutions. Since the legislation referred to institutions such as government laboratories, universities, medical societies, and philanthropic organizations, the Department of Health obviously had concerns about granting the authority for vivisection investigations directly to a commercial firm.[67]

The staff of the Merck Institute grew from just three in 1933 to twenty-one in 1938, and the number of scientific publications produced by the laboratory went from one in 1934 to sixteen in 1938. The early reports of the institute, as well as its publications, indicate that the laboratory was engaging in pharmacological research as well as testing compounds for their pharmacological properties and carrying out biological standardization of products. Molitor noted in his 1938 report that the requirement for premarket testing of new drugs for toxicity included in the 1938 Food, Drug, and Cosmetic Act would necessitate greater emphasis on toxicology on the part of the institute.[68] The major pharmaceutical firms were already carrying out some kind of testing of drug products on a voluntary basis, either in house or with the aid of outside consultants. However, the requirement that new drugs must comply with FDA safety regulations before being introduced onto the market created an increased need on the part of the pharmaceutical industry for the services of pharmacologists.

The report of the Merck Institute for 1935 provides an overview of the work of the laboratory in a typical year from this period. The total staff of the institute at this time (including janitors) was fifteen. Molitor admitted that he had had difficulty in hiring trained scientists, who tended to prefer working in an academic setting. He indicated that he had been successful, however, in training high school graduates, who pursued college studies at night, as technicians. The institute had worked on eighty-six different research problems in 1935, although many of these were narrowly defined projects. Molitor classified eleven of these problems as fundamental, originating in his laboratory. The rest involved the investigation of the therapeutic properties of new drugs or plants submitted to the laboratory or the testing of claims made by the discoverers of new pharmaceutical products. A total of 74 compounds were investigated, 30 of which were new synthetic chemicals, 10 of which were plants of tropical origin, and 34 of which were chemical modifications of known drugs. Of the synthetic chemicals, 14 originated in the research laboratories of Merck and 16 were submitted by outside scientists. The vast majority of these compounds (95 percent) exhibited no therapeutic value and work on them was quickly abandoned, but research was continued on those substances that seemed most promising as therapeutic agents. In addition to this research, the laboratory performed a relatively small number of routine assays and seventy-one biological standardizations.[69]

Although Molitor did not achieve quite the same level of recognition that Chen did among American pharmacologists, he was a highly qualified scientist who was respected by his peers. Richards, for example, thought very highly of him.[70] Chauncey Leake, professor of pharmacology at the University of California, San Francisco, wrote to Molitor in 1936 to congratulate him on the fine work of his laboratory. Leake added: "I was skeptical that you would have the opportunity for such work at the Institute. My first impressions were that you would be required chiefly to carry through routine work of such nature as to prevent any fundamental studies from going on."[71]

Although the entry of scientists of the caliber of Chen and Molitor into the pharmaceutical industry helped to improve the image of industrial pharmacologists among their academic colleagues, it was not until 1941 that pharmacologists employed by drug firms were accepted into membership in their national professional society.

The Bias against Industrial Pharmacologists

Readers familiar with Sinclair Lewis's classic novel *Arrowsmith*, published in 1925, will probably recall the character of Max Gottlieb, the idealistic immunologist who serves as a father figure to the young Martin Arrowsmith. At one point in the narrative, Gottlieb, who has always criticized the commercialism of certain large pharmaceutical firms, is forced for financial reasons to work for one of these companies. When the news of this situation reached the laboratories of great scientists around the world, "sorrowing men wailed 'How could old Max have gone over to that damned pill-peddler?'"[72]

Although this incident is taken from a work of fiction, it reflects a real-life attitude on the part of many academic scientists toward their industrial colleagues in this period and beyond. Nowhere is this suspicion of scientific work carried out in industrial firms better illustrated than in the case of American pharmacology. Drug industry pharmacologists were actually banned from membership in the national society for American pharmacologists from its founding in 1908 until 1941.

There were few pharmacologists associated with industry in the United States in 1908, yet the founders of the American Society for

Pharmacology and Experimental Therapeutics (ASPET) were apparently concerned enough about a potential threat from this quarter to insert the following two clauses into the new organization's constitution:

> No one shall be admitted to membership who is in the permanent employ of any drug firm.
> Entrance into the permanent employ of a drug firm shall constitute forfeiture of membership.[73]

These steps were taken, in the words of the society's council, "in order to avoid every external influence which would be inimical to the scientific interests of pharmacology."[74]

It is not clear who first proposed the ban on industrial pharmacologists, but the committee which drafted the constitution consisted of Abel and three of his former associates at Johns Hopkins: Reid Hunt (chairman), Arthur Loevenhart, and Albert Crawford.[75] Whoever suggested the ban, it seems to have met with the general approval of the founders of the society. Available correspondence and other records indicate that there was no debate over adopting the ban, though there was significant discussion about other membership matters, such as whether or not to admit clinicians who were not actually engaged in pharmacological research (see chapter 6).[76] Apparently no one saw fit to challenge the prohibition against industrial pharmacologists, and a serious movement to change this rule did not begin for about another decade.

This prohibition against industrial scientists appears to be unique among American professional scientific societies.[77] No doubt anti-industry bias existed on the part of academic scientists in other societies, but it was not carried to the extreme of explicitly singling out industry scientists for exclusion from membership. The American Chemical Society, for example, had developed significant ties with industry by the beginning of the twentieth century. The first specialized division organized by this society was the Division of Industrial and Engineering Chemistry in 1907, reflecting the large number of industrial chemists in the society. Several of the society's presidents in the period from 1880 to 1920 were associated with the chemical industry.[78]

Both the American Physiological Society and the American Society of Biological Chemists had a close relationship with the pharmacology society, and both included industrial scientists as members. The American Physiological Society admitted pharmacologist Elijah Houghton of the pharmaceutical firm Parke, Davis and Company as a member in 1901. An associate of Abel's at Johns Hopkins, Thomas Aldrich, was admitted to the physiologists' society in 1895 and did not have to relinquish his membership when he moved to Parke-Davis a few years later. In 1916, Aldrich, still at Parke-Davis, was admitted to membership in the American Society of Biological Chemists.[79]

Why did the pharmacologists resist admitting industrial scientists into their national society when their colleagues apparently did not hesitate to do so? What were the external influences "inimical to the scientific interests of pharmacology" that they were trying to avoid? Motivation is usually difficult to establish, and the early leaders of the society did not leave a clear record of justification for their action. The existing evidence allows the following suggestions of at least some of the concerns that motivated American pharmacologists in this matter.

During the first decade of the twentieth century, when the society was founded, the American drug industry had a somewhat suspect reputation. Thousands of patent medicines of a dubious nature flooded the market, and patent medicine quackery, brought to public attention by muckraking journalists of the Progressive Era, was one of the factors that led to the passage of a national pure food and drug act in 1906. Although the more legitimate drug firms tried to distance themselves from the patent medicine promoters, they were not completely successful in lifting the cloud of suspicion that hung over the industry as a whole.[80]

Even the so-called ethical firms sometimes engaged in practices that pharmacologists considered objectionable. For example, Abel complained that his name had been used on occasion without his permission in drug advertisements or on drug labels. In a 1910 letter to a colleague, he warned: "Even reputable firms will do things that tend to damage men."[81] Five years later he expressed this skeptical view about the advertising practices of drug manufacturers: "It is well known that the advertisers of drugs and medicines have often failed to confine their statements to actual facts and have yet to get the confidence of our profession."[82]

The traditional opposition of the medical community to patenting medical discoveries, reflected already in the Code of Ethics of the American Medical Society at its founding in 1847, probably influenced the views of many pharmacologists toward research in commercial firms.[83] Most of the first generation of American pharmacologists were trained as medical doctors, for there were no graduate programs in the subject in the United States (see chapter 4). Even those who studied the subject abroad, like Abel, usually received the M.D. degree. Seventeen of the eighteen founders of the American Society for Pharmacology and Experimental Therapeutics possessed medical degrees. By contrast, only fourteen of the twenty-nine founding members of the American Society of Biological Chemists (1905) had M.D. degrees, and six of them were also founders of ASPET who in most cases considered their profession as pharmacology rather than biochemistry. Certainly only a relatively small proportion of the members of the American Chemical Society had M.D. degrees at the time. On the other hand, the American Physiological Society, which did not ban industry scientists, was also heavily medical in its membership.[84]

Pharmacologists may have been especially sensitive, relative to other scientists, about commercial influences on their work. It was the work of the pharmacologist, rather than that of the chemist or biochemist, that would determine at the experimental level the therapeutic potential and toxicity of a new drug. Academic pharmacologists were concerned that their industrial colleagues were perhaps subject to pressures from their employers to emphasize positive results and downplay negative results. For example, Robert Hatcher of Cornell expressed concern in a 1919 letter that "nearly all workers in commercial houses deplore the limitations of their work due to the pressure for financially productive results, and to the necessity of avoiding publications that are inimical to financial interests." He added that one "need hardly ask proof that pressure is often put on investigators to supply desireable results."[85]

Torald Sollmann of Western Reserve University indicated that the founders of ASPET believed that a pharmacological society was "obliged to take these peculiar precautions, because otherwise it would be exposed to peculiar dangers."[86] Similarly, Samuel Meltzer of the Rockefeller Institute argued that the *Journal of Pharmacology and Experimental Therapeutics*, founded by Abel in 1909, had to be more careful about drug advertisements than, for example, a journal of morphology. He pointed out that many people would interpret an advertisement in the pharmacological journal as implying authoritative approval of a drug.[87]

Fears were also expressed that industrial pharmacologists might use the forum provided by the society's annual meetings to extol the virtues of the products marketed by their employers. Reid Hunt, for example, expressed to Abel his concern that "the scientific meetings of the Society might become an opportunity for the reading of papers on drugs being exploited, or to be exploited, commercially."[88] The society was so concerned about this potential problem that soon after it became a part of the newly created Federation of American Societies for Experimental Biology in 1912, a motion was passed to ask that the federation not transfer any paper to the ASPET program without the explicit consent of the secretary of the society. The main purpose of this resolution was to prevent the appearance on the program of papers of a "commercial nature."[89]

John Abel was sensitive, as might be expected, about possible exploitation of the *Journal of Pharmacology and Experimental Therapeutics* for commercial purposes. The first paper from an industrial laboratory did not appear in the journal until the sixth volume (1914), and there were few such papers before 1925. On the other hand, most American pharmaceutical firms were not carrying out much research that would have been suitable for publication in the journal in the first quarter of the century. In 1918 Francis Stewart of the Mulford Company claimed that Abel had recently indicated a greater willingness to receive papers from industrial sources, although several years later Abel was still expressing concern that he had to be on his guard about criticism in publishing papers from manufacturing firms. He commented with respect to two of these papers submitted that year that they "might give the impression of not being sufficiently impartial from a scientific point of view" and that "some might get the impression that there is an advertising element in the papers." His main concern in the case of these two papers appears to have been the use of the trade names of the drugs involved. Abel felt that the trade names should be deleted entirely, or at most mentioned in brackets (following the chemical names) once or twice near the beginning of the paper, but not in the title or in any of the tables.[90]

One must also recall that in the early years of the society, American pharmacology was still struggling to become a legitimate academic discipline. Pharmacology was trying to escape the role assigned to materia medica, which was often viewed as essentially a handmaiden to therapeutics. John Abel and other leaders in the field emphasized that pharmacology was a basic biological science, related to but distinct from physiology.[91] Research carried out in pharmaceutical firms was considered to be largely of a practical or applied nature, and not contributing to the development of the fundamental science. Abel once explained to a colleague why he himself would not consider working on any problem suggested by a pharmaceutical firm: "Usually, problems of this nature could be worked out very well in the laboratories of the firms since they almost always concern questions of what I might call applied pharmacology. A pharmacologist of any training or ability should have so many problems of his own awaiting solution that he should not spend his time on matters of little theoretical importance for his science."[92]

Struggling to establish their discipline as an independent, basic science, the practitioners of pharmacology were especially anxious to avoid any taint of commercialism. Abel was so scrupulous on this point that when he was elected as the society's first president in 1908, he resigned from a special commission investigating the safety of saltpeter as a food additive. Although the commission was organized through the University of Illinois, it was funded in part by the American Packers Association. As the first president of an organization which banned industry pharmacologists from membership, Abel was concerned that his connection with the commission might be misunderstood, especially when he learned that rumors were circulating that he was "in the employ of the meat firms."[93]

In less than a decade, Abel began to soften his views on the question of industry pharmacologists. In early 1916, he wrote to a colleague in London that at the recent meeting (December 1915) of ASPET in Boston he had sounded out some of the older members, such as Samuel Meltzer and Torald Sollmann, about admitting pharmacologists in drug firms, such as Elijah Houghton, to membership in ASPET. He noted, however, that his colleagues were opposed to this step, believing that the time was not ripe for such an action. There was a feeling, he added, that "the drug house will not play 'fair' and will 'do us' at every opportunity."[94]

The issue was soon raised again, this time by Arthur Loevenhart of the University of Wisconsin. In 1918 Loevenhart discussed the question with Abel and, after receiving his support, submitted an amendment the following year to delete the membership restriction from the constitution. The amendment did not come up for a vote until the 1920 meeting, and it was soundly defeated.[95] Abel apparently still had mixed feelings about the issue, admitting to a colleague after the meeting that he was less inclined to favor the amendment than he had been two years earlier.[96]

For the next two decades the issue remained controversial, periodically resurfacing to plague the society. During this period, the proponents of changing the rule against industrial pharmacologists were unable to obtain the necessary four-fifths vote at an annual meeting to change the constitution on this point. Sentiment to eliminate the restriction continued to grow, however, and culminated in the successful vote of 1941.

There were probably two major factors that contributed to the movement in the 1920s and 1930s to eliminate the ban against industrial pharmacologists. The first of these factors was the increase in the amount and quality of research being carried out by American pharmaceutical companies in the period between the two world wars. Many pharmaceutical companies established research facilities in the post–World War I period, and some of the more prestigious companies began to become involved in basic research to some extent. As the image of research in the pharmaceutical industry improved, the stigma of industrial pharmacology decreased. As respected scientists such as K. K. Chen at Lilly and Hans Molitor at Merck followed in the footsteps of the fictional Max Gottlieb and joined the staff of pharmaceutical companies in the 1920s and 1930s, the pressure to change the society's constitution increased.[97]

In arguing the case for such a change, Abel wrote to Reid Hunt in 1927 that the large drug firms now had a better attitude toward research than they had had thirty years earlier.[98] In a letter to Sollmann in the same year, he noted that an increasing number of good pharmacologists either were not finding, or were not interested in, academic positions and were pursuing careers with the larger pharmaceutical companies. Noting that he had originally been opposed to admitting industrial pharmacologists when the society was founded, Abel added: "But times have changed and I wonder if we should not change with them."[99]

A second factor to be considered was the increasing involvement of academic pharmacologists as consultants or in collaborative research agreements with the drug industry in this period.[100] For example, Loevenhart and later his successor at Wisconsin, Arthur Tatum, became involved in collaborative research on organic arsenical drugs with Parke, Davis and Company beginning in the 1920s.[101] In the early 1930s, University of Pennsylvania pharmacologist Alfred Newton Richards became a consultant to Merck on a regular basis and assisted that firm in developing an in-house program of pharmacological research.[102]

These consulting or collaborative arrangements were approached cautiously at first. Several collagues, for example, wrote to Abel for counsel before undertaking such projects, seeking his opinion about the propriety of accepting payment from a pharmaceutical firm for performing professional service.[103] Such arrangements became increasingly common and acceptable after World War I, and no doubt influenced the views of at least some pharmacologists about their industrial colleagues.

Even the traditional opposition on the part of many physicians and biomedical scientists to patenting medical discoveries began to erode in this period. By the mid-1930s at least a dozen universities were administering patents on medical discoveries by their faculty, further blurring the line between science and commerce.[104]

Those who supported changing the ASPET constitution to admit industrial pharmacologists argued that it was unnecessary to have a specific prohibition against these individuals. The society's constitution and bylaws, it was claimed, provided adequate safeguards against the admission of unqualified members. Those who failed to meet the standards of the society would be rejected, and any member who acted unethically or unprofessionally in some manner could be expelled under another provision of the constitution.[105]

Loevenhart complained that some, like Sollmann, criticized the low standards of pharmacological work in industry but stood in the way of a major reform that might help to elevate these standards. Admitting industrial pharmacologists into ASPET would improve the chances of pharmaceutical firms to hire first-rate scientists, and company pharmacologists would benefit from interaction with their academic colleagues.[106]

Opponents of the change, however, were not satisfied with these arguments, and continued to express concern that industrial pharmacologists might eventually dominate the society and bend it to the needs of industry.[107] Robert Hatcher emphasized that the ideals of even the best scientists would gradually be broken down "by constant association with those who are in business with its insistent demand for financial success."[108] Some members tried to work out a compromise, whereby industry pharmacologists would be admitted as a new class of "associate members," but without the privilege of voting. But even this step went too far for some hard core opponents of change, and some of those who favored eliminating the membership restriction were concerned that this procedure would still mark their industrial colleagues as second-class citizens. The compromise effort never succeeded, and the issue remained unresolved.[109]

Some pharmacologists accepted the restriction on membership gracefully. For example, when K. K. Chen joined the staff of Eli Lilly and Company in 1929, he submitted his resignation to ASPET, expressing "a desire to comply with the ethics of the Society and leave it in good standing."[110] Others employed by industrial firms were understandably disturbed by the restriction on membership. For example, in 1928 pharmacologist David Macht of Hynson, Westcott and Dunning wrote to Simon Flexner complaining about "the terrible and unjust discriminations made by other scientists more particularly medical men and pharmacologists against anyone connected with a commercial concern."[111] He was especially angered by what he called the "preposterous provision" in the constitution of the pharmacological society which excluded those employed in drug firms from membership.[112] British pharmacologist Henry Dale, who had worked for a pharmaceutical firm early in his career, would have sympathized with Macht on this point, for in 1933 he wrote to an American colleague that he regarded the attitude of ASPET toward industrial pharmacologists as "a piece of silly hypocrisy and pedantic snobbery."[113]

Although the rule remained in the constitution throughout the 1930s, at least one point was clarified during this decade. The question arose as to whether the phrase "in the permanent employ of a drug firm" included a paid consultation arrangement with a pharmaceutical company on a long-term basis. Pharmacologists had been consulting with drug firms before the 1930s, but the number of such arrangements increased, and some of these involved extensive consultation over a long period of time. The matter seems to have come to a head when A. N. Richards wrote to the council of ASPET on 4 April 1935, explaining that he had been acting as a paid consultant for Merck for three years, and that he felt it was his duty to bring this arrangement to the council's attention because of the rule denying membership to those in the "permanent employ" of drug firms.[114]

The council considered Richards's letter at its 1935 meeting, and agreed that the rule needed to be clarified with respect to consulting arrangements. A special committee was therefore established to study the problem, and in the meantime Richards was told that the council did not deem that the arrangement he had with Merck violated the constitution.[115] It was recognized that by this time quite a few members were consulting with pharmaceutical firms.[116]

The committee, chaired by William deBerniere MacNider of the University of North Carolina, and including Abel as one of its members, recommended clarifying the two clauses in the constitution barring those "in the permanent employ of a drug firm" by adding the phrase "other than in the capacity of a consultant." Consulting arrangements would thus be explicitly excluded from the rule. They also proposed changing the term "drug firm" to "any organization concerned with the manufacture or sale of medicinal products." A majority of the members present at the 1936 annual meeting of ASPET (twenty-seven of forty-four) favored the amendment, but it did not receive the four-fifths majority needed for it to pass.[117] The same amendment was introduced again at the 1937 meeting, and this time it passed, although some members expressed concern about the advisability of passing an amendment "legalizing" consultation.[118] Meanwhile, there was no change in the status of pharmacologists whose sole or primary employer was a pharmaceutical company.

With the establishment of the Squibb Institute for Medical Research in 1938, its newly appointed chief pharmacologist, Harry Van Dyke, tried a different approach to retaining his membership in the society. Van Dyke pointed out that the Squibb Institute had been established for basic research, that it had its own board of scientific directors, and that it was relatively independent of the Squibb Company. He argued that he was therefore not really in the employ of a drug firm.[119] But the society's council refused to accept this argument. One officer commented: "Suppose Van Dyke would come out with a paper condemning, in no uncertain terms, one of E. R. Squibb and Son's preparations. Van Dyke would lose his job. In other words, this means that Van Dyke is dependent upon E. R. Squibb and Sons for his livelihood."[120] In any case, the council felt that Van Dyke should not be treated differently from Chen, Molitor, and other industrial pharmacologists.[121]

Nevertheless the pressure to alter the constitution continued. In November 1940, twenty-four distinguished members of the society submitted another amendment to eliminate the ban on membership for industrial pharmacologists. The list of names included several who had been long-time opponents to amending the constitution for this purpose, such as Torald Sollmann and C. W. Edmunds.[122] It is not clear why these staunch foes of the amendment decided to change their position at this particular time, but certainty their switch played a key role in the eventual victory of the pro-amendment movement.

On 17 April 1941, the seventy-two members present at the annual business meeting of ASPET unanimously approved amending the constitution to delete the restriction against industrial scientists, thus ending thirty-three years of a discriminatory policy.[123]

The improved image of industry science as pharmaceutical companies became more seriously involved in fundamental research, the employment of distinguished pharmacologists by industry, and the increasing involvement of academic scientists as consultants to industry all contributed to the eventual change in ASPET policy toward membership for industrial pharmacologists. The efforts of reputable drug firms to distance themselves from the manufacturers of quack patent medicines and increasing government regulation of the drug market may have also been factors in making the climate more favorable for the acceptance of industry pharmacologists by ASPET.

In spite of, or perhaps because of, increasingly friendly relations between academics and the pharmaceutical industry over the past half-century, the considerations that motivated the founders of ASPET to institute their membership ban on industrial pharmacologists have not disappeared. The close ties that have developed between industry and academia in recent times have caused renewed worries that the former may come to dominate the latter, and that science may become commercialized in the process. As John Swann noted in his book on the history of this interaction with respect to the pharmaceutical industry in the United States: "Universities, industry, and the public now have to decide how much collaboration is desirable for their needs; how much profit and impartiality they are willing to sacrifice; and which is the best possible course to satisfy the public good."[124]

CHAPTER SIX

The Professionalization
of a Discipline

The Creation of a National Society

The consolidation and "professionalization" of a discipline requires institutional structures such as specialized academic departments, societies, and journals to help define the field, including setting (and defending) its boundaries. As Robert Kohler has pointed out with respect to the development of various biomedical disciplines in America around the beginning of the twentieth century: "New journals and professional societies and insistence on specialized credentials sharpened disciplinary boundaries and made poaching more difficult."[1]

We have discussed the emergence of pharmacology departments in American universities, and how they replaced the traditional materia medica programs, as well as the development of the science in nonacademic settings. This chapter focuses largely on the creation of two other mechanisms by which pharmacologists established and shaped their field as an independent discipline in the United States: a national society and a journal for the profession. Once again, John Abel played a pivotal role in these developments, as he had in forging an academic tradition of experimental pharmacology in this country.

Before turning to the founding of the pharmacological society and journal, it is relevant to first briefly examine Abel's earlier experience as an organizer in the field of biochemistry. For, in spite of his academic position as a pharmacologist, it was actually in his other scientific love, biological chemistry, that Abel first decided to establish a journal and a society. But, whereas in pharmacology, the founding of the society preceded that of the journal, in biological chemistry, the order was reversed.

The question arises as to why Abel elected to devote his early efforts to creating a journal of biochemistry rather than one in pharmacology. This is particularly puzzling in light of the fact that the

cofounder and coeditor of the publication, Christian Herter, also held
an academic position as a pharmacologist, at Columbia University (see
chapter 4). Biochemistry was probably no more firmly established as
a discipline in the United States than pharmacology at the time. Both
Herter and Abel had broad interests in biomedical science, however,
and were committed to the application of chemistry to medical and
biological research. Contributors to and readers of the *Journal of
Biological Chemistry* were not intended to come soley from the then
small community of biochemists in America. Rather, as announce-
ments for the journal emphasized, the journal's scope would be broad,
including such fields as bacteriological chemistry, plant chemistry,
and clinical chemistry. Its pages were to be open to zoologists, botanists, physiologists, pathologists, pharmacologists, bacteriologists,
clinicians, and organic chemists, as well as biochemists, as long as the
work was of a chemical nature. The journal was to reflect the growing
interest in "chemical research in the elucidation of general biological
and medical problems." Abel and Herter most likely believed that a
broad-based journal such as this would have more support than one
focused more specifically on the interests of one disciplinary group,
and would serve their commitment to the chemical approach.[2]

Abel first approached Herter with the idea of a journal of biological
chemistry in the spring of 1903. Herter indicated that a similar idea
had been in his mind, and that he believed there would be enough
good American research devoted to chemical problems in physiology
and pathology to support such a publication.[3] Formal steps toward
establishing such a journal were not taken until 1905, when Abel wrote
to twenty-one colleagues inviting them to serve as collaborating editors
and to submit papers for the journal. Abel and Herter served as coeditors of the new publication, with A. N. Richards, then working with
Herter (see chapter 4), serving as managing editor. The journal was
incorporated in New York, with the three editors, along with Reid
Hunt (see chapters 4 and 5) and Edward K. Dunham (professor of
pathology at the University and Bellevue Hospital Medical College of
New York University) serving as directors. The first issue of the new
journal appeared in October 1905.[4]

The American Society of Biological Chemists, organized in 1906
with Abel again taking the lead, was as broad-based as the journal.
Efforts were made to recruit members from the various biological
sciences, as well as from chemistry and medicine. Kohler has estimated
that only about one-third of the eighty-one founding members were

physiological or medical chemists. Although some members of the American Physiological Society had expressed concerns that the new journal and society might splinter the physiological field and jeopardize the survival of their own organization and publication, both societies and journals survived and flourished.[5] Years later Abel recalled that even before the founding of the *Journal of Biological Chemistry* in 1905, he had concluded that the American Physiological Society should have one or more daughters, noting that: "From a close study of her case I came to the conclusion that she was pregnant and did not know it."[6]

It is clear that Abel was planning the formation of a national professional society for pharmacologists even before the biochemical society was formally established. Although the circular letter sent out by Abel on 13 December 1906 concerning the biochemistry organization makes no reference to a pharmacological society, Abel most likely added a postscript to the copies of the letters that went to certain of his colleagues, for several of them made reference in their replies to a possible pharmacology group.[7] Torald Sollmann, for example, said that Abel could count on his support in all of his plans and added: "of course, I am more interested in the Assoc'n of Pharmacologists, but both are very necessary."[8] Robert Hatcher stated that he hoped Abel's views concerning the formation of a pharmacological society would be carried into effect, and George Wallace indicated his support for such an association.[9]

William Gies, in discussing the plans for the imminent founding of the biochemical society, also referred to the efforts: "looking to the formation of a pharmacological society, which you have communicated confidentially."[10] Abel chose not to try to establish both societies at once. He may well have limited the discussion of the pharmacological society in 1906 out of a realistic concern that such an action would only intensify the fears of those who saw the founding of the biochemistry society as the beginning of the end of the American Physiological Society. He did not wait long after the establishment of the biochemical society, however, before taking active steps to create an analogous society for pharmacology.

The first meeting of the biochemical society, after its organizational session, was a special one held in conjunction with the Congress of American Physicians and Surgeons in Washington, D.C., in May 1907.[11] Abel wrote to Sollmann in January 1907 stating that he hoped to present plans for a journal of pharmacology "before the members of the proposed Society" at the May meeting; this suggests that Abel was contemplating founding the pharmacological society at that time.[12] The association was not organized in Washington, however, and in December Abel wrote to several colleagues suggesting that they meet to organize the new society at the joint meeting of the American Physiological Society and the American Society of Biological Chemists in Chicago in December 1907.

There was some difference of view among those consulted as to whether or not to begin organizing the society in Chicago. Some believed that since a majority of the prospective members lived in the East, and most of these would not be at the meeting, it would be better to wait a year until the next combined meeting of the two established societies, which was to be held in Baltimore. Others favored making a start on organizing the society in Chicago. Abel decided to wait until he got to Chicago to make a decision. In the end, he was very busy with the biochemistry meeting and relatively few pharmacologists were on hand, so no action was taken regarding the new society.[13] Shortly after the Chicago meeting he wrote to Sollmann:

My idea of the matter now is that we should make all efforts to organize here in Baltimore next winter at the time of the meetings of all of the societies. It is high time that we started a society. Our subject is suddenly getting popular. Twenty years ago there was very little interest taken in it. Fifteen years ago I wrote on the subject trying to arouse the interest of physicians but the thing would not go. Now that a man like our friend Simmons [presumably George Simmons, editor of the *Journal of the American Medical Association*] is showing some interest in the subject, the ordinary medical schools are waking up. Last year there were about ten places for pharmacologists, mostly associate Professorships, and no good men or at least not enough for the places. It would do some of the younger men a lot of good, I know, to belong to a society of specialists who are enthusiastic and willing to discuss their papers.[14]

In December 1908, Abel sent an invitation to a select group of people to attend a meeting to organize a national pharmacological society. The meeting was to be held in the lecture room on the third floor of the Johns Hopkins Medical School building on 28 December, at the time of the annual meeting of the physiology and biochemistry societies. Abel's announcement indicated that a number of pharmacologists had already signified their approval of such a plan and had expressed the view that the proposed society would further the development of pharmacology and experimental therapeutics. He reminded his colleagues "that Pharmacology and Experimental Therapeutics are the only departments of scientific medicine that still remain without an organization and a journal."[15]

On 28 December 1908, eighteen men met in the pharmacology lecture room of the Johns Hopkins Medical School to establish the American Society for Pharmacology and Experimental Therapeutics. Of this group, eleven were employed by universities, five worked for the federal government, and two were based at a private research facility, the Rockefeller Institute for Medical Research. One member, Velyien Henderson of the University of Toronto, was Canadian; all the others were Americans. Seventeen of the founders possessed M.D. degrees, and sixteen of them were also members of the American Physiological Society.

Not surprisingly, Abel was elected president of the new organization, and his protégés Reid Hunt (United States Public Health Service) and Arthur Loevenhart (University of Wisconsin) were named secretary and treasurer, respectively. Samuel J. Meltzer (Rockefeller Institute), Torald Sollmann (Western Reserve University), Charles W. Edmunds (University of Michigan), and Albert C. Crawford (United States Department of Agriculture) were selected to be members of the association's council, along with the officers. The council was charged with preparing a constitution for the government of the society.[16]

The name of the new society occasioned some discussion. According to Torald Sollmann, the group wanted to use the name "American Pharmacological Society," but there already existed an association with a very similar name, the American Pharmacologic Society. This group, which had been founded by Francis E. Stewart (see chapter 5) in 1905, was not designed to promote the interests of professional pharmacologists, but had as its object the promotion of "progress in pharmacologic science, and in the useful arts of pharmacy, pharmacognosy, pharmacodynamics and drug therapeutics." Its membership was open to a wide variety of individuals, including physicians, pharmacists, chemists, botanists and any other persons "dependent upon the pharmacologic arts, and the manufacture of food-products." The organization, and Stewart's plan to have it raise revenues by carrying out scientific investigations on food and drug products for manufacturers for a fee, does not appear to have ever really gotten off the ground.[17]

A more significant question than the use of the noun or the adjective to designate pharmacology in the society's name was the addition of the phrase "and Experimental Therapeutics." Experimental therapeutics was a term popularized by the noted German scientist Paul Ehrlich, who had criticized pharmacology for concentrating on the investigation of the effects of drugs on healthy animals. Ehrlich emphasized the need to produce diseases experimentally in animals and then study the action of drugs against these diseases, a field that he called experimental therapeutics. Ehrlich's work and ideas had already attracted significant attention by 1908, when the society was founded, and were soon to become even more visible through his receipt of the Nobel Prize in Physiology or Medicine in 1909 (for his work in immunology) and the announcement of his discovery of the antisyphilitic Salvarsan in 1910. The term *experimental therapeutics* was almost certainly included in the name of the society, as Sollmann has claimed, to emphasize the relationship of pharmacology to Ehrlich's work, and particularly to his chemotherapeutic research. Probably stung by Ehrlich's criticism of their field, pharmacologists were quick to embrace chemotherapy as a part of their discipline.[18]

Much of the early discussion concerning who should be admitted to membership in the society centered on the question of how far to go in accepting clinicians involved in some kind of therapeutic research. There was, on the one hand, a desire to attract respected clinicians who would enhance the prestige of the new society, but at the same time there was a concern about the danger of the organization losing sight of its principle focus, experimental pharmacology. Torald Sollmann and Samuel Meltzer, both more involved in clinical medicine than many of their pharmacological colleagues, favored a broader view of membership that would admit more clinicians. Meltzer, for example, argued for a liberal spirit with respect to admitting good clinicians, while maintaining high scientific and moral standards.[19]

Albert Mathews (University of Chicago), on the other hand, was concerned about "getting pharmacology too much under the wing of the clinicians." Mathews was head of the Department of Physiology's Laboratory of Bio-Chemistry and Pharmacology, and the holder of a Ph.D. degree rather than a medical degree. Favoring the laboratory over the clinic, he feared that too practical an approach to the subject stifled "all growth and breadth."[20]

I believe that the greatest danger in the formation of the society will come from the clinical side. I think it advisable to move with great

caution in admitting clinicians until the science is pretty well established. There are always so many men so short sighted as to wish a
science to develop with its practical applications always the main thing
in it, whereas experience has so abundantly demonstrated that no
science can develop properly unless the practical applications are
regarded as secondary not primary.[21]

Carl Alsberg of the Bureau of Plant Industry, United States Department of Agriculture, worried that the generous admission of clinicians would defeat what he believed was one of the main purposes
of the society: "to stamp [the] subject as an independent discipline"
rather than as a branch of internal medicine. He felt so strongly about
this issue that at the organizational meeting of the society he had
opposed adding "Experimental Therapeutics" to the organization's
title. His fear was that such an expansion of the scope of the group
might mean that anyone connected with internal medicine could be
regarded as eligible for membership.[22]

Charles Edmunds proposed a compromise, based on a suggestion
by his colleague at the University of Michigan, bacteriologist Frederick
Novy. Rather than admitting clinicians on the same basis as those who
made pharmacology or experimental therapeutics their life's work,
they could be made associate members. This idea did not meet with
much favor, however, and was not adopted. Reid Hunt wondered
about how many clinicians would want to be classified as pharmacologists or experimental therapeutists in any case.[23]

Clearly the founding members of the new society were struggling
to shape their identity. The old fears about pharmacology, like its
predecessor materia medica, serving as only a servant to the therapeutics of clinical practice were still close to the surface. Pharmacologists were not unique in feeling this tension between the clinic and
the laboratory in a period when laboratory science was transforming
medicine. For example, Gerald Geison has discussed the efforts of
physiology to proclaim itself a separate discipline (and not a mere
handmaiden of medicine) and the conflict that resulted at times between physician and scientist. And Russell Maulitz has pointed out
the tensions that developed between laboratory science and clinical
medicine with respect to bacteriology in the late nineteenth and early
twentieth centuries. All of these sciences struggled to be independent
of medicine, but, in the words of Geison (speaking of physiology), the
prospects of the new disciplines "remained closely bound up with the
destinies of medicine and medical education."[24]

In addition to grappling with the relationship of their field to clinical medicine, pharmacologists were also concerned with its status vis-à-vis sister biomedical sciences such as biochemistry and bacteriology. There were scientists whose primary allegiance was to other disciplines but who did carry out some research of a pharmacological nature and therefore could be considered eligible for membership. William Gies, for example, was invited to join, although he held the chair of physiological chemistry rather than pharmacology at Columbia University, because, as Hunt noted, "there was a good deal of pharmacological work being done there." Some members saw a danger in admitting too many of these "outsiders." Sollmann worried, for example, that the new association might tend to lose its identity as a pharmacological society if it admitted too many bacteriologists. He suggested limiting membership to bacteriologists who were making the study of immunity their life's work (presumably because of the relation of immunity to experimental therapeutics). Meltzer argued that there were too many investigators in the field of immunity to admit them all. As in the case of the clinicians involved in therapeutic research, it was suggested that some kind of associate membership could be created for biomedical scientists whose main field was not pharmacology. This time the proposal came from Sollmann, who thought it might be wise to consider scientists who worked in fields where pharmacology was purely incidental as "other collaborators." He added: "If we do not draw this line, we might as well take in all the physiologists, pathologists, bacteriologists and chemists and thus lose our individuality." Again, the proposal for two classes of membership was not adopted by the society.[25]

In all, thirty-four members were elected to the society in 1909, and these were considered charter members along with the original eighteen men who had founded the organization.[26] There were no women among the charter members. Less than half of the new group could be classified as pharmacologists. The others by and large were prominent clinicians such as George Washington Crile (a surgeon with an interest in physiology) and George Dock (who had just moved as professor of medicine from Michigan to Tulane) and noted bacteriologists such as Frederick Novy and Theobald Smith. Although the founders of the society clearly wished to represent pharmacology as a distinct discipline, they were also obviously motivated by a desire to expand their size to a more respectable level and to include distinguished individuals whose membership would reflect credit on the organization (even though they were not pharmacologists).

Another requirement of membership was that the individual must have published "a meritorious investigation in pharmacology or experimental therapeutics," and must also be "actively engaged in research in these fields." The fields of pharmacology and experimental therapeutics were broadly interpreted in some cases. The society was interested, however, in limiting its membership to those who had at least made some kind of published research contribution. An early draft of the constitution, in fact, specified "two meritorious investigations," but the final version reduced the requirement to one. There was room for disagreement, of course, about what constituted a "meritorious investigation."[27] As discussed in the previous chapter, there was one group of pharmacologists which was ineligible for membership, regardless of how numerous or meritorious their contributions might be, namely those scientists who worked for the drug industry.

Following the organizational meeting in Baltimore, the society convened for the first annual meeting in Boston in December 1909, at the time of the meeting of the American Physiological Society. A constitution was adopted and dues were set at one dollar per year. A total of twenty-two members were present at the Boston meeting, and the scientific program included eighteen papers and demonstrations.[28]

Beginning with just over fifty members in its first full year (1909), the society grew relatively slowly. Its membership did not reach one hundred until 1921 and did not exceed two hundred until the year of Abel's death (1938). These figures reflect the fact that even after pharmacology had established its place as a distinct discipline worthy of its own specialized academic chairs, society, and journal, its growth was slow and steady rather than explosive. At the end of the Second World War, membership was still only about three hundred, in contrast with some four thousand members today.[29]

A Journal for the Field

Abel recognized early on that American pharmacology needed its own journal as well as a society in order to help promote the discipline. Just as Abel had in mind eventually founding a society for pharmacology at the time that he was establishing one for biochemistry, he seems to have had similar plans with respect to journals in the respective fields. Christian Herter recalled that he and Abel had intentionally excluded pharmacology from the title of the *Journal of Biological Chemistry* when it was founded in 1905 so that the field would be left open for a pharmacological journal. By 1907 Abel was corresponding with Herter about the prospects of starting a pharmacology journal.[30]

When Abel circulated his call for a meeting to organize a pharmacological society in November 1908, he included a reference to the desirability of establishing a journal for the field as well. As in the case of the *Journal of Biological Chemistry*, Abel created a corporation to run the new *Journal of Pharmacology and Experimental Therapeutics*. In 1909 a Journal of Pharmacology and Experimental Therapeutics Society was established and incorporated in Baltimore to own and operate the journal. The incorporators were Abel, Christian Herter, and Carl Voegtlin (who was working in Abel's laboratory at the time). The three incorporators served as the board of directors of the journal society as well as its only initial members. Other members could be added if elected by the board, which also elected the officers and board members. In other words, the three incorporators (and, for all practical purposes, Abel as the editor) completely controlled the journal.[31]

When it came to getting the journal published, Abel turned to Waverly Press of the Williams and Wilkins Company, the Baltimore firm which was then printing the *Journal of Biological Chemistry*. This latter journal had been consistently losing money in its early volumes, but was able to survive through substantial personal subsidies from Christian Herter. Abel was not in a position to provide the kind of financial support that Herter could, nor could Herter be called upon to subsidize another journal. Abel therefore proposed to Edward Passano, president of Williams and Wilkins, that the company serve not only as printer, but also as publisher, of the new journal. The company, in other words, would assume the financial risks involved in the venture. A contract for publication of the journal was signed with Williams and Wilkins on 16 March 1909, marking the beginnings of the firm's extensive involvement as a publisher of scientific journals.[32]

The announcement issued to publicize the new journal emphasized the value of having its own journal for the discipline of pharmacology:

> Investigators in the various biological and medical sciences, no less than those who are merely students in these fields, find it greatly to their convenience that researches in each department of knowledge should be published in a separate journal. Up to the present time

pharmacologists and students of experimental therapeutics have published their work in journals devoted to other experimental sciences, but the activity of investigators in these fields would now appear to justify the existence of a separate journal.[33]

Pharmacology had thus justified, in Abel's view, its place as a "department of knowledge," worthy of its own specialized journal. The announcement went on to state that the pages of the journal would be open not only to "professional pharmacologists and workers in experimental therapeutics," but to scientists from other fields wishing to offer papers that had a close relationship to pharmacological or therapeutical questions. (Note Abel's use of the term "professional pharmacologists.") The notice also indicated that at least six issues of the journal would be published annually, with the first to appear by 1 May 1909 (although it was not actually published until June).

Abel served as editor of the publication and the initial announcement listed thirteen associate editors. Ten of these individuals can probably be labeled as "card-carrying" pharmacologists: A. C. Crawford, C. W. Edmunds, R. A. Hatcher, C. A. Herter, R. Hunt, A. S. Loevenhart, S. J. Meltzer, F. Pfaff, A. N. Richards, and T. Sollmann. It is true that Herter was as much of a biochemist or pathologist and Meltzer as much of a physiologist as they were pharmacologists, but they were significantly involved in pharmacological activities. One could perhaps also consider adding David L. Edsall, then professor of therapeutics and pharmacology at the University of Pennsylvania, to this list, although he was certainly seen by Abel and others as more of a representative of experimental therapeutics. The other two associate editors, Simon Flexner, director of the Rockefeller Institute for Medical Research, and G. N. Stewart, professor of experimental medicine at Western Reserve University, also represented experimental therapeutics (and, in Flexner's case, the relationship of bacteriology and immunology to therapeutics).[34]

The first volume of the journal (1909–10) contained a total of thirty-three papers. Not surprisingly, by far the greatest number of papers (twenty-four) came from academic institutions. Six papers came from government agencies, four of these from Hunt's laboratory in the United States Public Health and Marine Hospital Service and two from Crawford's laboratory in the United States Department of Agriculture's Bureau of Animal Industry. The remaining three papers were from a private foundation laboratory, the Rockefeller Institute

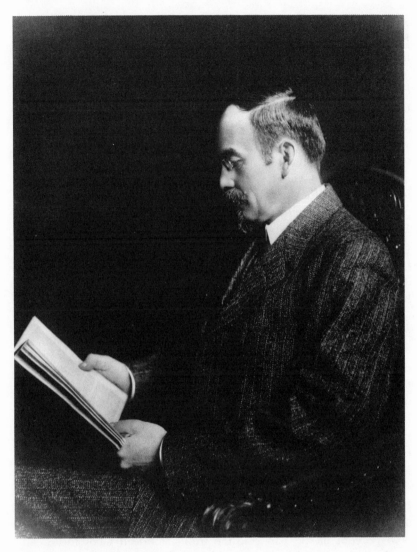

John J. Abel, founder and first editor of the Journal of Pharmacology and Experimental Therapeutics.

Courtesy of the National Library of Medicine.

for Medical Research. There were no papers from industrial laboratories, which is not surprising given the relative paucity of pharmacological research in American firms at the time and the suspicion with which the new society viewed industry pharmacologists (see chapter 5).

As might be expected, the largest university contributor was Johns Hopkins, with 9 papers of the 24 that came from academia. Other universities contributing papers to the first volume of the journal were Michigan (4), Columbia (2), Toronto (2), Western Reserve (2), Wisconsin (2), Cornell (1), Missouri (1), and Virginia (1). These were all universities that had active pharmacology programs by 1909. The two papers from V. E. Henderson's pharmacological laboratory at Toronto were the only papers from outside the United States. Just over half of the academic papers (13) came from departments of pharmacology (one of which was a combined department of pharmacology and physiology). Three other papers were coauthored by workers from Abel's pharmacology laboratory, along with someone from one of the Johns Hopkins clinical departments. The remaining 8 papers (one-third of the total) had no connection with pharmacology departments, but came from departments of clinical medicine or of other laboratory sciences (such as bacteriology and physiology). All of the academic papers, however, came from departments in medical schools.[35]

This mix of papers in the first volume was not atypical of the general distribution of papers over the journal's first three decades, for the greater part of which Abel served as editor. The major changes over that time period were that some papers began to come from industrial laboratories (the first in 1914) and academic departments outside of the medical school, and that the number of foreign papers began to increase significantly after 1912, when Abel made an arrangement with the British (as discussed below). The proportion of papers from government and private foundation laboratories was also lower over the entire period than it was during the first year.

It is instructive to examine in more detail the figures for the first three decades, from 1909 through 1938 (the year in which Abel died, although he gave up editing the journal in 1932). Over this period, 80.5 percent of the papers came from American laboratories, and another 19.5 percent from foreign (including Canadian) institutions. An analysis of the American papers provides some evidence of where pharmacological research was carried out in the United States (at least in so far as it is reflected in the pages of the national professional journal for pharmacologists).

Academic institutions dominated the picture, with 81.3 percent of the papers coming from universities. The rest of the papers were roughly evenly divided between industrial firms (4.6 percent), government agencies (7.4 percent), and private, noncommercial laboratories such as the Rockefeller Institute (6.8 percent). About two-thirds of the academic papers involved pharmacology departments, 61.6 percent of them coming solely from such departments and another 6.2 percent jointly from pharmacology and another department. Slightly more than one-quarter (27.5 percent) were from medical school departments other than pharmacology. Only a small percentage (4.7 percent) came from university departments outside of the medical school. Pharmacological research in America thus continued to be centered in academic institutions, and especially in medical schools, through the 1930s.

During the journal's first five years (1909–13), more than one-quarter of the papers (18; 28 percent), came from Johns Hopkins University. No other institution came close to matching this output. Other universities that contributed an average of at least one paper per year during this period were Wisconsin (8), Michigan (6), Western Reserve (6), Northwestern (6), and Washington University (5). A total of fourteen academic institutions had papers published in the journal in these formative years. By the 1930s, active research programs had been established in many more universities, and the field was not as dominated by one or even several institutions. In the period 1935–39, for example, the journal published papers from forty-two different universities. Johns Hopkins University contributed only 4 percent of the papers during this five-year span, and the largest university contributor (Stanford) accounted for only 12 percent of the total.[36]

In 1912 the journal took on more of an international flavor with the formal involvement of British pharmacologists. The British did not have their own society or journal in the field at the time, as pharmacology remained a part of physiology much longer in Great Britain than in the United States. The British Pharmacological Society was not founded until 1931, and the first issue of the *British Journal of Pharmacology and Chemotherapy* was not published until 1946.[37] Thus in 1911, Arthur Cushny, then professor of pharmacology at University College, London (see chapter 3), suggested to his friend John Abel the establishment of an arrangement by which the *Journal of Pharmacology and Experimental Therapeutics* could serve as a major publication medium for British as well as American pharmacologists. Abel had considered naming some British pharmacologists to the journal's editorial board when it was first established, but Herter advised him that there was no point in this as the British would no doubt continue to publish their work at home (presumably in physiology or medical journals).[38]

There was widespread enthusiasm on the part of the journal's editorial board for a joint agreement with their British colleagues. Arguments in favor of such a plan were that it would help to insure both the financial stability of the journal and the quality of its contents. Since the journal had indeed been having financial problems, the prospect of increased subscriptions no doubt enhanced the appeal of Cushny's proposal. Monetary considerations aside, however, the board members also believed that such a move would also increase the influence and prestige of the publication. An arrangement with the British might crowd out some of the work of American pharmacologists, wrote Robert Hatcher, but he felt that such fears did not deserve consideration. The agreement that was established involved the appointment of ten British scientists to the journal's Board of Associate Editors, including a joint (with Abel) editor-in-chief, a position originally filled by Cushny. This joint arrangement lasted until the British pharmacologists founded their own journal in 1946.[39]

Although Abel did not keep systematic files on the journal, letters in his general correspondence give some idea of his editorial style. He tended to be generous in accepting papers, especially in the journal's first decade or so when the pressure for space was not so great. Papers were apparently generally not refereed, especially if they came from the laboratories of members of the editorial board or other established pharmacologists. In the 1920s, Abel began to complain about the length and number of papers that were being submitted, and the backlog that was developing. The British collaborators and some of Abel's American colleagues urged him to be more selective in accepting papers and more severe in editing them, a strategy for which Abel had little taste. He defended himself by saying that he had refused papers when he could, but felt this could not very well be done with papers from members of the relatively large editorial board. He also argued that the British were able to deal with manuscripts in a more critical spirit and with more authority than it was generally possible for American editors to exercise (an assumption that seems unwarranted). Instead, Abel tried to get Williams and Wilkins to increase the number of volumes per year from two to three. In 1922 he even suggested to one colleague that he might have to consider excluding papers from "outsiders" (i.e., those not on the editorial board), an extreme step that was never taken.[40]

Hatcher suggested that Abel could depersonalize the issue by submitting the papers to a board, but Abel was afraid that such an editorial committee would still make bitter enemies by just doing its job. As he indicated to one colleague, he also favored a "one man policy" of running a journal. He reluctantly agreed, however, to try to institute, as he expressed it to Carl Alsberg in 1922, "a more stringent policy and boldy refuse to accept the weaker sort of papers." As the 1920s progressed, Abel does seem to have turned more frequently to referees to critically review papers, but he was not always satisfied with the results. He complained to one colleague that whenever he gave a paper to a referee, he got into difficulties. Abel did not enjoy arbitrating disagreements between authors and referees.[41]

Although editorial standards for the journal may have tightened over the 1920s, there was obviously still a good deal of "cronyism" at work as Abel hesitated to offend established scientists. In 1928, for example, he wrote to one colleague: "You know that I am a very busy man and that I rarely read the articles sent to me when they come from the laboratories of my associate editors." When associate editor Robert Hatcher complained about a paper from one of his students that was rejected based on a referee's report, Abel apologized and offered to publish the paper anyway, even if the referee's suggestions for revision were not incorporated. In another example, in 1930 Abel responded to a query about the status of two manuscripts submitted from the laboratory of a distinguish French scientist by stating that "it goes without saying that any paper with Fourneau's name on it would be accepted without question."[42]

Two other interesting editorial policies relate to vivisection and to the acceptance of advertising. Obviously vivisection played an important role in pharmacological research, and most pharmacological papers published in the journal involved some animal experiments. Abel of course supported animal experimentation, but as a journal editor he could not completely ignore antivivisection and animal welfare sentiments. For example, in 1929 he refused a paper partly on the grounds that it involved brain surgery on animals that were not anesthetized. After conferring with surgical colleagues at Johns Hopkins, who advised him that anesthesia probably could have been used in the procedure without affecting the results, Abel concluded that it would have been "disadvantageous" for him as an editor to publish the paper. He wrote to the author: "I hope that you will find an editor who is willing to take the risk of publishing it even though you have operated on animals without the use of an anesthetic."[43]

Abel was not, in general, opposed to experimentation on unanesthetized animals. In fact, in 1928 he wrote to a colleague: "I have been preaching a doctrine for many years that anesthetics should be avoided in our pharmacological experimentations wherever possible."[44] Abel took this position because, as stated in a paper from his laboratory, "anesthesia is known to disturb seriously the metabolic processes in dogs, as well as other species of laboratory animals." About the same time that he rejected the paper mentioned above, he published papers from his laboratory and from the pharmacological laboratory at the University of Iowa which involved the study of the effects of drugs and of heat and cold on unanesthetized dogs. Both of these papers claimed that anesthesia would have interfered with the experiments, and neither paper involved surgical procedures carried out without anesthesia. Abel presumably believed that the absence of anesthesia in these experiments was more justifiable and less controversial than in the case of the brain surgery work reported in the rejected manuscript.[45]

In 1929 Abel also expressed concerns about another paper which he feared would cause the antivivisectionists to attack both the *Journal* and the institution where the research had been carried out, the Hygienic Laboratory. He was particularly worried about the research protocols described in one of the tables, which summarized the toxic effects of inhaled chloroform on dogs which had previously been given alcohol. He suggested to the author, Sandford Rosenthal, that Rosenthal might speak to his supervisor, Carl Voegtlin, about this point, although Abel thought it likely that "the protocols must stand." Voegtlin suggested changing the terms used in describing the toxic symptoms in the dogs "so as to make them sound less harsh to the anti-vivisectionists." It is not known whether Voegtlin's suggestion was adopted, but the description of the symptoms of the dogs in the published paper included terms that were not likely to appease antivivisectionists, such as "extremely sick," "vomiting," "does not eat," and "found dead."[46]

Abel was not unique among editors of biomedical journals in his concerns about the antivivisectionists. Susan Lederer has discussed how editorial concerns about antivivisection in the 1920s through the 1940s altered the descriptions and illustrations of laboratory procedures involving live animals in the pages of the *Journal of Experimental Medicine*. Peyton Rous, editor of this journal, and his staff read manuscripts carefully with an eye to preempting conflicts with antivivisectionists. They substituted words that they considered to be impersonal medical descriptions for those terms that might highlight animal suffering (such as "fasting" for "starving" or "hemorrhaging" for "bleeding"), suggested avoiding photographs of the entire animal when its condition was "unsightly" or it was undergoing an operation, and took other steps designed to avoid providing ammunition to the antivivisectionists.[47]

With respect to another editorial policy, the *Journal of Pharmacology and Experimental Therapeutics* did include advertising during its early history, but Abel closely controlled the acceptance of advertising copy. He insisted that all advertisements be reviewed by him. Abel would have preferred that the journal not accept any advertisements from pharmaceutical firms, but financial conditions made him loath to press Williams and Wilkins too hard for such a policy. Instead he encouraged advertisements that merely provided a general statement of the kinds of products produced by a company, without "laudatory comments." If advertisements for proprietary drugs were to be accepted, these had to be limited to products that were approved by the American Medical Association's Council on Pharmacy and Chemistry. In spite of these policies, oversights sometimes occurred. To Abel's chagrin, for example, two advertisements were published in 1916, without his approval, that referred to products that had not been approved by the council. The situation was especially embarrassing because after Abel had apologized to George Simmons of the American Medical Association for the first of these transgressions, the second offending advertisement appeared while Simmons was reviewing the copy for it at Abel's request.[48]

In 1929 Abel also refused to accept a cigarette advertisement. He indicated to Williams and Wilkins that he would prefer to limit advertisements to chemical firms, book publishers, instrument makers, and the like. In any case, he did not feel that it was appropriate to accept an advertisement from a firm that had gotten itself into trouble recently for advising young women to smoke their cigarettes instead of eating sweets in order to keep their "fashionable slim figures."[49]

Abel continued to edit the journal until 1932, the year in which he retired from his university position. Upon retiring at the age of seventy-five, an autonomous Laboratory for Endocrine Research was created for Abel at Johns Hopkins so that he could continue his research as a professor emeritus. Although he directed the work of the laboratory, he devoted his remaining years to an entirely new field of research for him, the study of tetanus toxin. This work was supported by funding from outside agencies, especially the Carnegie Corporation.[50]

In his retirement years, Abel's contributions were recognized by several honors. For example, he served as president of the American Association for the Advancement of Science in 1932–33, delivering his presidential address on the subject of poisons and disease at the association's annual meeting in Boston on 17 December 1933. Abel was awarded the George Kober Medal of the Association of American Physicians in 1934, and on the last day of his life he received notification of his election as a foreign member of the Royal Society of London.[51]

Abel's last years were clouded by the illness of his wife, who became an invalid about 1930. She suffered several apoplectic strokes, resulting in the paralysis of the left side of her body and some impairment of her mental faculties in 1935. In the final years of her life, Mary Abel required full-time nursing care.[52] She died on 20 January 1938 at the age of eighty-seven. Seven years earlier, John Abel had recalled his first meeting with Mary in a letter addressed to her from aboard a ship carrying him to Europe: "You are not old to me sweetheart; I still see you as you were, when you came into the dining room of the hotel at La Porte, so many years ago, and bowled me over when you turned your fine eyes on me as you were placed at my side at dinner!"[53]

John Abel survived his wife by just a few months. He continued to work actively in his laboratory right up to the end of his life. Two or three weeks before his death, Abel developed a cough which led to suspected bronchopneumonia. Although he curtailed his activities and allowed himself to be examined at home by a colleague, Abel resisted entering the hospital. Finally, however, he was admitted to the Johns Hopkins Hospital, where he died on 26 May 1938, a week after his 81st birthday, of a coronary thrombosis. Just a few hours before his death, he discussed plans for the continuation of his research on tetanus toxin with one of his laboratory associates.[54]

As for the *Journal of Pharmacology and Experimental Therapeutics*, when Abel retired in 1932 he was succeeded as editor by the man who also followed him in the pharmacology chair at Johns Hopkins, E. K. Marshall, Jr. Marshall had obtained a Ph.D. in chemistry from Johns Hopkins in 1911, and then obtained his M.D. there in 1917, while also working in Abel's laboratory. After wartime work in the Chemical Warfare Service (chapter 5) and a brief period as professor of pharmacology at Washington University in St. Louis, Marshall returned to Johns Hopkins as professor of physiology in 1921. Upon Abel's retirement, Marshall moved to the chair of pharmacology.[55]

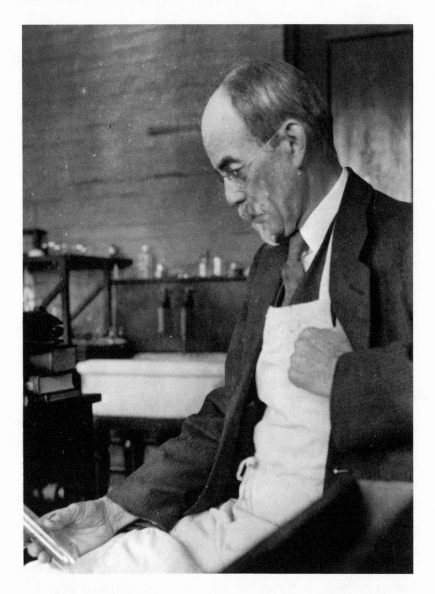

John J. Abel in his laboratory at the Johns Hopkins University, 1926.
Courtesy of the National Library of Medicine.

At about this time, Abel also took steps to transfer the ownership of the journal from his private corporation to the American Society for Pharmacology and Experimental Therapeutics. Although Abel provided space in the pages of the journal for the abstracts of papers given at the society's meetings, there was no official connection between the two. A feeling grew among some pharmacologists that the journal should be recognized in some way as the official organ of the society. Neither Abel nor Marshall had any objection to the society's actually taking over the responsibility for the journal if that seemed desirable, and discussions on this point began in 1932.

The five-year contract then in effect with Williams and Wilkins for publication of the journal ran through 16 March 1934, and this seemed to Abel to be an appropriate time for transfer of ownership to take place. A special session was set up on 9 April 1933, during the society's annual meeting in Cincinnati, to discuss the transfer of the journal and a new arrangement with Williams and Wilkins. The society wanted to take over the ownership of the journal from Abel, but discussions with Edward Passano, president of Williams and Wilkins, at this meeting and the next day failed to achieve a satisfactory agreement on a publishing contract. Passano, who had developed a good working relationship with Abel, was concerned that the society might eventually decide to act as its own publisher and exclude his company entirely. He believed that Williams and Wilkins deserved some equity in the publication for its efforts and risks over the years. He tried to negotiate an arrangement where the society would agree to cover any deficits or pay the company a percentage of the receipts in lieu of equity if the society desired to take over the publication of the journal at the end of the contract period. Passano returned to Baltimore without a contract agreement.

Abel left the society's meeting early and rode back on the train with Passano. During the course of that train ride, he apparently convinced Passano to drop any demands on the society that it guarantee to cover any deficits or compensate the publisher for services rendered. Abel took the next train back to Cincinnati with a letter from Passano to this effect, arriving in time to present it at the last business session of the society on April 12. The offer to accept ownership of the journal from Abel was then accepted and a new contract was established with Williams and Wilkins. The first American professional society and journal in the field of pharmacology were thus firmly united.[56]

Epilogue: An Established Discipline

By the time of the First World War, American pharmacologists had their own national society and journal. In addition, the subject was firmly established at a significant number of the country's most reform-minded medical schools and had begun to find a place in government and commercial laboratories.

During the interwar period, the discipline continued to expand in size and influence. Pharmacologists began to be employed by other academic health sciences programs, such as schools of pharmacy, a trend that intensified after the Second World War. The number of pharmacology graduate programs, which had their tentative beginnings at a few schools before the end of the First World War, also increased in the 1920s and 1930s, although doctoral training in pharmacology still remained on a relatively small scale.

The specialized expertise of pharmacologists came to be recognized in various other ways over the first four decades of the twentieth century. Pharmacologists such as Charles Edmunds, Robert Hatcher, Reid Hunt, and Torald Sollmann played an important part in the work of professional bodies such as the American Medical Association's Council on Pharmacy and Chemistry and the United States Pharmacopeial Convention's Revision Committee. Their services as expert witnesses in court were utilized by regulatory agencies such as the Food and Drug Administration. Several pharmacologists, such as John Abel, Reid Hunt, William deBerniere MacNider, and Alfred Newton Richards were elected to the National Academy of Sciences, beginning with Abel in 1912.

At the time of John Abel's death in 1938, the subject that he had nurtured from its American infancy had thus achieved a certain maturity as an independent scientific discipline. In spite of this obvious progress, however, many pharmacologists remained concerned about the state of their field on the eve of the Second World War. In 1969 Maurice Seevers, writing when he was professor of pharmacology at the University of Michigan, looked back at the 1930s as dark days for pharmacology, a period when its survival as an independent discipline was at stake. Although Seevers may have been presenting an extreme view, others worried during the 1930s that pharmacology was not advancing, or perhaps was even backsliding. Pharmacologists of the period complained that their subject was not accorded quite the same respect as some of the preclinical sciences, and a 1940 report of the American Medical Association showed that eighteen of the country's sixty-six four-year medical schools still did not have a separate department of pharmacology. In these institutions, pharmacology was combined in a department with another subject, generally physiology or biochemistry, and such joint departments were rarely headed by pharmacologists.[57]

Writing in 1940, Alan Gregg of the Rockefeller Foundation argued that improving the status of pharmacology in American medical education should be one of the goals of medicine for the upcoming decade.

> Relative to the value of therapeutic discoveries in the past thirty years, and relative to the potentialities of chemotherapy, and relative to the size of the drug industry in the United States, the support and esteem "enjoyed" by pharmacology in the medical schools is absurd. And the scarcity today of pharmacologists qualified for teaching posts, governmental appointments or industrial positions is lamentable— or exciting, if you don't think it is too late. Here is a subject for a whole series of papers, and study of a large number of personal communications I have elicited convinces me that it is high time that American medical schools increase their attention to pharmacology *in esse* and *in posse*.[58]

If there were concerns for pharmacology's future at the close of the 1930s, the revolution in drug therapy over the past half-century has largely laid these to rest. Beginning with the introduction of antibiotics into therapeutics during World War II, and extending to recent drug discoveries to combat diseases such as AIDS and cancer, the ability of the physician to treat diseases with pharmaceutical agents has been enormously increased. As historian James Harvey Young has noted: "The quarter century following the enactment of the Food, Drug and Cosmetic Act of 1938 witnessed a revolution in the drugs which doctors prescribed for ailing patients. So vast was it in scope, so significant in repercussions, this revolution ranks as one of the major events in medical history."[59]

The expansion of the pharmaceutical industry and of the governmental regulation of drugs have provided greatly increased employment opportunities for pharmacologists. The need for health professionals to keep up with the explosive growth in knowledge related to the increasing array of pharmaceutical products has also strengthened the case for pharmacology in the curricula of students of pharmacy, nursing, dentistry, and veterinary medicine, as well as in medical schools. By 1988 there were graduate programs for the training of pharmacologists in some 188 schools of medicine, pharmacy, and veterinary medicine in the United States.[60] Increasingly, pharmacologists hold Ph.D. rather than M.D. degrees; of forty-seven new regular members of the American Society for Pharmacology and Experimental Therapeutics in 1991, forty possessed a Ph.D. degree.[61]

A 1989 survey of the field showed that medical schools remained the largest employer of professional pharmacologists, employing 44 percent of those surveyed. The pharmaceutical industry was the second most common employer, with approximately 28 percent of the respondees working in this environment. Pharmacy schools were the third most common employer of professional pharmacologists with 6.5 percent, followed by federal government laboratories (National Institutes of Health; Alcohol, Drug Abuse and Mental Health Administration; Food and Drug Administration; Veterans Administration) with 5 percent. Another 2.4 percent were employed in schools of dentistry or veterinary medicine.

The field continued to be dominated by men, with only about 15 percent of the professionals being female. However, the percentage of pharmacologists who are women is likely to grow significantly in the future, because 41 percent of the students and 34 percent of the postdoctoral fellows responding were female. Minorities comprised 12.6 percent of the total respondees, the vast majority of them being Asian or Pacific Islanders (8.9 percent). African Americans and Hispanics each made up only 1.7 percent of the group.[62]

This survey provides a profile of those who practice pharmacology. But what of the science itself? Classical pharmacology has emphasized the investigation of the effects of substances on experimental animals, using the whole organism. In its early development, many of its leaders argued the need to withdraw from the bedside to the laboratory in the evaluation of the action of drugs. It was also pointed out that pharmacology could shed light on the action of toxins and other chemicals as well as medicinal agents. The basic science value of pharmacology was emphasized, without however denying its ultimate usefulness to therapeutics.

Although animal experimentation at the organism level still plays a major part in pharmacological investigation, traditional pharmacology has been buffeted from two opposing directions. On the one hand, concerns that it was becoming too remote from clinical medicine have led to the emergence of a subfield of clinical pharmacology. The beginning of clinical pharmacology as a distinct subject in this country is generally associated with the work of Harry Gold at Cornell University in the 1950s. In 1960 the *Journal of Clinical Pharmacology and Therapeutics* was established, and three years later the American College [later Society] of Clinical Pharmacology and Chemotherapy was created. This latter group merged with the much older American Therapeutic Society to form the American Society for Clinical Pharmacology and Therapeutics in 1969. Meanwhile, the American Society for Pharmacology and Experimental Therapeutics had established its own Division of Clinical Pharmacology in 1967. Clinical pharmacology began to compete for time with classical pharmacology in the medical curriculum.[63]

By definition, clinical pharmacologists are interested in research on human subjects rather than experimental animals. A practitioner in the field must have an M.D. degree, in contrast with the trend toward the Ph.D. in pharmacology as a whole. A specialty board to certify clinical pharmacologists (as exists in other medical specialties) was created in 1989, with the first examination taking place in 1991.[64] The relationship between clinical pharmacology and therapeutics is exceedingly close, and this subfield thus tends to pull the science of pharmacology closer to medical practice.

Pharmacology has also been pulled in the opposite direction, toward the cellular and molecular level, by the advent of molecular biology. Efforts to understand the action of drugs at a cellular level go back at least to the receptor theory developed by Paul Ehrlich in Germany and by John Newport Langley in England at the beginning of the twentieth century. A. J. Clark's refinement of receptor theory and efforts to quantify drug action in works such as his *The Mode of Action of Drugs on Cells* (1933) greatly stimulated interest in cellular pharmacology.[65] The pharmacologist traditionally served in the role of "critic," testing the safety and efficacy of substances isolated from natural products or synthesized in the laboratory. In recent decades, the elucidation of biochemical and physicochemical mechanisms by which drugs reach and act on the cell has led to a more "rational" pharmacology, with the pharmacologist playing a greater role in the development of "made-to-measure medicinal agents."[66] However, empirical approaches have continued to play a significant role in drug discovery, as exemplified by the large-scale screening processes for identifying useful antibiotics.

Watson and Crick's paper on the double helix structure of deoxyribonucleic acid (DNA) in 1953 ushered in the era of molecular biology, a development that affected all of biomedical science.[67] By the 1960s, pharmacologists such as Avram Goldstein were arguing that if the discipline were to survive and remain on the cutting edge of science it "had to embrace the molecular domain in a public way."[68] In 1965, the *Journal of Molecular Pharmacology* was founded, reflecting efforts to understand the action of drugs at the cellular and molecular level. Relations between the new molecular pharmacologists and more traditional pharmacologists were not always smooth, however, as reflected in the following statement by William Fleming:

> I am dismayed by the opinions I hear expressed by some cellular/molecular biologists and by some pharmacologists. Some, but certainly not all, cellular and molecular scientists show disdain for any research that is not done at the cellular or molecular level. On the other hand, some more traditional pharmacologists are digging in their heels and refusing to recognize the potential contributions that cell and molecular biology can make to our discipline.[69]

In spite of the tensions created by the forces pulling the field in different directions, the expansion of the traditional concerns of pharmacologists, extending all the way from the molecular level to the level of the whole human body, can be seen as making pharmacology stronger and more exciting. The coauthor of one textbook in the field pointed out that the first chapter of the work was entitled "Molecular Mechanisms of Drug Action" and the last "Drug Evaluation in Man," and he suggested that "from molecules to man" would be a good slogan for the field.[70]

Meanwhile, classical pharmacology has also come under attack as part of the resurgence of antivivisectionism in the form of the modern animal rights movement. The animal protection movement in the United States has grown dramatically since the publication of Peter Singer's *Animal Liberation* in 1975. Criticism of animal experimentation has helped to promote the search for alternative methods of research and testing, involving the use of tissue culture, microorganisms, computer simulation, and other non-animal methods. In recent years, journals and institutions devoted to the study of alternatives have been established.[71] Animal research has played such a dominant part in the development of pharmacology, as it has in related fields such as physiology, that any challenge to it is seen as a threat to the science itself. "Animal models and *in vivo* studies," argued the American Society for Pharmacology and Experimental Therapeutics in 1982, "are a condition *sine qua non* for pharmacologists."[72]

Yet it is unlikely that animals will be largely replaced in biomedical research and testing in the foreseeable future. And pharmacologists have a significant role to play in the development of alternative methods and the comparison of these to traditional animal models.

Classical pharmacology involving whole animal studies seems destined to continue to thrive, alongside the clinical and molecular approaches, for some time to come. William Fleming has argued that pharmacology will continue to exist as a broad discipline for at least two crucial reasons. First, "industrial developments of new therapeutic agents and vehicles cannot progress without scientists who understand and can carry out experiments at the organ and whole animal level." Second, "if we ever get away from a component of medical education delivered by faculty interested in the effects of drugs in the whole organism, we will be turning out physicians whose therapeutic knowledge is totally inadequate."[73]

Pharmacology has always been an interdisciplinary field, drawing upon various other disciplines to a significant extent for its methods, and often for recruits to its ranks. This broad basis, as suggested above, can be seen as a strength, even if it blurs the boundaries of the science. One prominent pharmacologist has commented about his discipline:

> Not biochemistry alone, nor physiology alone, nor chemistry alone, nor behavioral science alone, nor clinical investigation alone—but only all in concert can explain the actions of drugs, and can point the way to new drugs for the prevention and cure of disease. No field I know of can claim this rich a diversity, nor this direct a translation from basic discovery to applications for the good of humanity.[74]

John Abel would readily agree with this assessment. In 1924 he told Abraham Flexner that he had always maintained that the more varying types of pharmacologists in the discipline, the stronger it would be. "Let one pharmacologist be more of a chemist, another more of a physiologist, another more of a clinician."[75] Pharmacologists today are as diverse as Abel could have wished.

NOTES

Introduction

1. For recent definitions of *pharmacology* similar to this one, see Robert E. Stitzel, "Development of Pharmacological Thought," in Charles R. Craig and Robert E. Stitzel, eds., *Modern Pharmacology*, 2d ed. (Boston: Little, Brown, and Co., 1986), pp. 3–8, especially p. 3; John A. Bevan, "History and General Principles," in John A. Bevan and Jeremy H. Thompson, eds., *Essentials of Pharmacology: Introduction to the Principles of Drug Action* (Philadelphia: Harper and Row, 1983), pp. 2–7, especially p. 3.

2. On the history of the term *pharmacology*, see Melvin P. Earles, "Studies in the Development of Experimental Pharmacology in the Eighteenth and Early Nineteenth Centuries" (Ph.D. diss., University College, London, 1961), p. 11; Gert Preiser, "Zum Geschichte und Bildung der Termini Pharmakologie und Toxikologie," *Medizinhist. J.* 2 (1967): 124–34; James A. H. Murray, ed., *A New English Dictionary on Historical Principles* (Oxford: Clarendon Press, 1909), 7: 768; *Encyclopedia Britannica*, 11th ed. (Cambridge: Cambridge University Press, 1911), 21: 347.

3. Even the latest edition of the classic pharmacology textbook by Goodman and Gilman defines pharmacology in a broad sense and uses pharmacodynamics to refer to what is generally termed pharmacology by those in the field. See Leslie Z. Benet, Jerry R. Mitchell, and Lewis B. Sheiner, "General Principles," in Alfred Goodman Gilman et al., eds., *Goodman and Gilman's The Pharmacological Basis of Therapeutics*, 8th ed. (New York: Pergamon Press, 1990), pp. 1–2.

4. Carl F. Schmidt, "Pharmacology in a Changing World," *Ann. Rev. Pharmacol.* 23 (1961): 1–14 (the quotation is from p. 12).

5. Benet, Mitchell, and Sheiner, "General Principles," p. 1.

6. On the history of bioassay, see Peter Stechl, "Biological Standardization of Drugs Before 1928" (Ph.D. diss., University of Wisconsin–Madison, 1969).

7. On the receptor theory, see John Parascandola, "The Development of Receptor Theory," in M. J. Parnham and J. Bruinvels, eds., *Discoveries in Pharmacology* (Amsterdam: Elsevier, 1985), 3: 129–56.

8. For example, on the centennial of Abel's birth, a memorial volume was published under the title of *John Jacob Abel, M.D., Investigator, Teacher, Prophet, 1857–1938: A Collection of Papers By and About the Father of American Pharmacology* (Baltimore: Williams and Wilkins, 1957).

9. See, for example, Gerard Lemaine et al., eds., *Perspectives on the Emergence of Scientific Disciplines* (The Hague: Mouton, 1976).

10. Robert E. Kohler, *From Medical Chemistry to Biochemistry: The Making of a Biomedical Discipline* (Cambridge: Cambridge University Press, 1982); W. Bruce Fye, *The Development of American Physiology: Scientific Medicine in the Nineteenth Century* (Baltimore: Johns Hopkins University Press, 1987).

11. "Meeting Highlights," *Pharmacologist* 28 (1986): 19.

Chapter One   From Materia Medica to Pharmacology

1. John Lesch, *Science and Medicine in France: The Emergence of Experimental Physiology, 1790–1855* (Cambridge: Harvard University Press, 1984).

2. On the early history of studies on drugs and poisons, see Melvin Earles, "Early Theories of the Mode of Action of Drugs and Poisons," *Ann. Sci.* 17 (1961): 97–110; Melvin Earles, "Experimental Investigations of Viper Venom by Felice Fontana (1730–1805)," *Ann. Sci.* 16 (1960): 255–68; P. K. Knoefel, "Felice Fontana and Poisons," *Clio Med.* 15 (1980): 35–65.

3. Melvin Earles, "Early Scientific Studies on Drugs and Poisons," *Pharm. J.* 188 (1962): 47–51 (the quotation is from p. 49).

4. Lesch, *Science and Medicine*, p. 100.

5. Richard D. French, *Antivivisection and Medical Science in Victorian Society* (Princeton: Princeton University Press, 1975), p. 20.

6. This discussion of Magendie and the beginnings of experimental pharmacology is based primarily on Lesch, *Science and Medicine*, pp. 99–165; J. M. D. Olmsted, *François Magendie* (New York: Schuman's, 1944), pp. 35–44; Earles, "Early Theories."

7. On Bernard's pharmacological research, see J. M. D. Olmsted, *Claude Bernard, Physiologist* (New York: Harper and Brothers, 1939), pp. 185–95; J. M. D. Olmsted and E. Harris Olmsted, *Claude Bernard and the Experimental Method in Medicine* (New York: Henry Schuman, 1952), pp. 73–80, 96–97.

8. Olmsted and Olmsted, *Claude Bernard*, pp. 79–80. See also Claude Bernard, "Physiological Analysis of the Properties of the Muscular and Nervous Systems by Means of Curare," in Louis Schuster, ed., *Readings in Pharmacology* (Boston: Little, Brown and Co., 1962), pp. 75–81 (an English translation of a paper originally published in *Comptes Rendus des Séances de l'Académie des Sciences*, 43 [1856]: 825–29).

9. The discussion of the early teaching of medical botany or materia medica that follows is based largely upon A. G. Morton, *History of Botanical Science: An Account of the Development of Botany from Ancient Times to the Present Day* (London: Academic Press, 1981), pp. 115–25; C. D. O'Mal-

ley, "Medical Education during the Renaissance," in C. D. O'Malley, ed., *The History of Medical Education* (Berkeley: University of California Press, 1970), pp. 89–102; Richard Palmer, "Medical Botany in Northern Italy in the Renaissance," *J. R. Soc. Med.* 78 (1985): 149–57; Karen Reeds, "Renaissance Humanism and Botany," *Ann. Sci.* 33 (1976): 519–42.

10. Palmer, "Medical Botany," p. 149.

11. W. R. O. Goslings, "Leiden and Edinburgh: The Seed, the Soil and the Climate," in R. G. W. Anderson and A. D. C. Simpson, eds., *The Early Years of the Edinburgh Medical School* (Edinburgh: Royal Scottish Museum, 1976), pp. 1–18, see pp. 8–9.

12. Reeds, "Renaissance Humanism," pp. 533–39; Theodor Puschmann, *A History of Medical Education from the Most Remote to the Most Recent Times*, trans. and ed. Evan H. Hare (London: H. K. Lewis, 1891), pp. 408–9.

13. Allen G. Debus, "Chemistry, Pharmacy and Cosmology: A Renaissance Union," *Pharm. Hist.* 20 (1978): 127–37; L. W. B. Brockliss, "Medical Teaching at the University of Paris, 1600–1720," *Ann. Sci.* 35 (1978): 221–51; George Urdang, "How Chemicals Entered the Official Pharmacopeias," *Arch. Int. Hist. Sci.* 7 (1954): 303–14.

14. Puschmann, *Medical Education*, pp. 396–97; Charles Coury, "The Teaching of Medicine in France from the Beginning of the Seventeenth Century," in O'Malley, *Medical Education*, pp. 121–72, especially pp. 128–29; Theodor Billroth, *The Medical Sciences in the German Universities: A Study in the History of Civilization*, translated from the German (New York: Macmillan, 1924), p. 16. On Boerhaave, see the biography by G. A. Lindeboom in *Dictionary of Scientific Biography* (New York: Charles Scribner's Sons, 1970), 2: 224–28.

15. Erwin H. Ackerknecht, *Therapeutics from the Primitives to the 20th Century* (New York: Hafner Press, 1973), pp. 78–115; Oliver Wendell Holmes, "Currents and Counter-Currents in Medical Science," *Med. Commun. Massachusetts Med. Soc.* 9 (1860): 305–48 (the quotation is from pp. 337–38).

16. On Buchheim, see B. Holmstedt and G. Liljestrand, eds., *Readings in Pharmacology* (Oxford: Pergamon Press, 1963), pp. 76–80; Gustav Kuschinsky, "The Influence of Dorpat on the Emergence of Pharmacology as a Distinct Discipline," *J. Hist. Med.* 23 (1968): 258–71; E. R. Haberman, "Rudolf Buchheim and the Beginning of Pharmacology as a Science," *Ann. Rev. Pharmacol.* 14 (1974): 1–8; Marianne Bruppacher-Cellier, *Rudolf Buchheim (1820–1879) und die Entwicklung einer experimentellen Pharmakologie* (Zurich: Julius Druck, 1971). The quotations from Buchheim's *Beiträge* are taken from the English translation in Holmstedt and Liljestrand, *Readings*, p. 79.

17. On Schmiedeberg, see Holmstedt and Liljestrand, *Readings*, pp. 80–87; Kuschinsky, "Influence of Dorpat," pp. 267–69; Jan Koch-Weser and

Paul J. Schechter, "Schmiedeberg in Strassburg, 1872–1918: The Making of Modern Pharmacology," *Life Sci.* 22 (1978): 1361–72.

18. Quoted from Oswald Schmiedeberg, *Elements of Pharmacology*, translated from the German by Thomas Dixon (Edinburgh: Young J. Pentland, 1887), p. v.

19. Ibid., pp. 1–12.

20. On the development of pharmacology in the German-speaking universities, see Kuschinsky, "Influence of Dorpat"; Holmstedt and Liljestrand, *Readings*, pp. 103–10, 122–26, 147–50; Jost Benedum, "Vom Giessener pharmakologischer Institut unter Rudolf Buchheim und Karl Gaehtgens (1867–1898)," *Medizinhist. J.* 15 (1980): 103–19; Edith Heischkel, "Schauplätze pharmakologischer Forschung und Lehre im Jahre 1866," *Medizinhist. J.* 1 (1966): 110–17.

21. David L. Cowen, "Materia Medica and Pharmacology," in Ronald L. Numbers, ed., *The Education of American Physicians: Historical Essays* (Berkeley: University of California Press, 1980), pp. 95–121; on Morgan and the College of Philadelphia, see pp. 95–96 (the quotation is from p. 97).

22. Ibid, p. 97.

23. Ibid, p. 99.

24. Ibid., pp. 100–105 (the quotation is from p. 105).

25. Torald Sollmann, "The Early Days of the Pharmacological Society," in *Essays in the History of Pharmacology* (Memphis: Department of Pharmacology, University of Tennessee, 1963), pp. 126–36 (the quotation is from p. 129.

26. H. M. Bracken, *Outlines of Materia Medica and Pharmacology: A Textbook for Students* (Philadelphia: P. Blakiston, Son, and Co., 1895).

27. W. Bruce Fye, *The Development of American Physiology: Scientific Medicine in the Nineteenth Century* (Baltimore: Johns Hopkins University Press, 1987), pp. 54–55.

28. On Mitchell, see ibid., pp. 54–91.

29. For biographical information on Wood, see the article on him by Glenn Sonnedecker in the *Dictionary of Scientific Biography* (New York: Charles Scribner's Sons, 1976), 14: 495–97; George B. Roth, "An Early American Pharmacologist: Horatio C Wood (1841–1920)," *Isis* 30 (1939): 37–45; G. E. de Schweinitz, "Memoir of Dr. H. C. Wood," *Trans. Coll. Phys. Philadelphia* 3d ser., 42 (1920): 155–65; Hobart Amory Hare, "Horatio C. Wood, the Pioneer in American Pharmacology," ibid., pp. 170–74; Horatio C. Wood, Jr., "Reminiscences of an American Pioneer in Experimental Medicine," ibid., pp. 197–234. The comment about Wood's middle initial by his son appears in Roth, "Early American Pharmacologist," p. 37.

30. H. C. Wood, "Hyoscine.—Its Physiological and Therapeutic Action," *Ther. Gaz.* 9 (1885): 1–10.

31. H. C. Wood, *A Treatise on Therapeutics, Comprising Materia Med-*

ica and Toxicology, with Especial Reference to the Application of the Physiological Action of Drugs to Clinical Medicine (Philadelphia: J. B. Lippincott, 1874). See especially the preface (pp. 5–10) for Wood's views on the value of animal experiments with drugs.

32. Wood, "Reminiscences," p. 216.

33. Ibid., pp. 216–17.

34. "Dr. Wood's Bibliographical Record," *Trans. Coll. Phys. Philadelphia* 3d ser., 42 (1920): 242–57.

35. Alan Mason Chesney, *The Johns Hopkins Hospital and the Johns Hopkins University School of Medicine: A Chronicle* (Baltimore: Johns Hopkins Press, 1943–58), 1: 76–79 (the quotation is from p. 79).

36. H. N. Martin, "The Study of the Physiological Action of Drugs," *Trans. Med. Chir. Fac. Maryland* 88 (1885): 79–92 (the quotation is from pp. 81, 90). I wish to thank A. McGehee Harvey for calling my attention to this paper.

37. J. S. Billings to D. C. Gilman, 15 May, 29 September 1884, Founding Documents, Alan Mason Chesney Medical Archives, The Johns Hopkins University, Baltimore.

38. On Brunton, see the article by William Bynum in *Dictionary of Scientific Biography* (New York: Charles Scribner's Sons, 1970), 2: 547–48.

39. J. S. Billings to D. C. Gilman, 15 May, 29 September 1884 and Matthew Hay to J. S. Billings, 11 May 1884, Founding Documents, Chesney Archives. See also Simon Flexner and J. T. Flexner, *William Henry Welch and the Heroic Age of American Medicine* (New York: Viking Press, 1941), pp. 490–91.

40. J. S. Billings to Matthew Hay, 11 October 1884; Memorandum of Proposals Made to Dr. Hay by the Executive Committee, 1 December 1884; D. C. Gilman to Matthew Hay, 4 December 1884; Matthew Hay to D. C. Gilman, 9 February 1885; Minutes of the Executive Committee, 2 March 1885; Founding Documents, Chesney Archives.

41. Because this case is of interest from the point of view of the full-time issue, it receives significant attention in Chesney, *Johns Hopkins*, 1: 86–89.

42. Matthew Hay to D. C. Gilman, 14 August 1886, Founding Documents, Chesney Archives.

43. On the financial difficulties of the university at this time, see Chesney, *Johns Hopkins*, 1: 95–97.

Chapter Two   The Education of a Medical Scientist

1. These details on Abel's family and early home life are largely derived from materials gathered by Dr. E. M. K. Geiling, a protégé of Abel who had intended to write a biography of him. The materials now comprise record group 8 of the John Jacob Abel Papers, Alan Mason Chesney Medical Ar-

chives, the Johns Hopkins Medical Institutions, Baltimore. See especially a 7-page untitled, undated typescript (presumably prepared by Geiling) on the Becker and Abel families and copies of letters from Frank Schaefer to Geiling, 9 May 1956 and 13 February 1958. For general biographical information on Abel, see William deBerniere MacNider, "Biographical Memoir of John Jacob Abel, 1857–1938," *Biog. Mem. Natl. Acad. Sci.* 24 (1947): 231–57 (includes a bibliography of Abel's publications); Carl Voegtlin, "John Jacob Abel, 1857–1938," *J. Pharmacol. Exp. Ther.* 67 (1939): 373–406; *John Jacob Abel, M.D., Investigator, Teacher, Prophet, 1857–1938: A Collection of Papers by and about the Father of American Pharmacology* (Baltimore: Williams and Wilkins, 1957); special issue of the *Bull. Johns Hopkins Hosp.* (vol. 101, no. 6, December 1957); Charles E. Rosenberg, "John Jacob Abel," *Dictionary of Scientific Biography* (New York: Charles Scribner's Sons, 1970), 1: 9–12.

2. E. M. Brown to John Abel, 7 July 1878 and John Abel to Mary Hinman, 22 October 1882, Abel Papers, record group 1; Paul Boston to E. M. K. Geiling, 26 April 1956 and Howard Hill to Geiling, 29 November 1955, Abel Papers, record group 8.

3. John Abel to Mary Hinman, undated [June 1881] and 22 June 1881, Abel Papers, record group 1.

4. John Abel to Mary Hinman, 28 and 31 June 1881, Abel Papers, record group 1.

5. John Abel to Mary Hinman, 24 July 1881, Abel Papers, record group 1.

6. John Abel to Mary Hinman, 28 June 1881, Abel Papers, record group 1.

7. John Abel to Mary Hinman, 13 August 1881, Abel Papers, record group 1.

8. John Abel to Mary Hinman, 6 August 1881, 7 July and 6 September 1882, Abel Papers, record group 1.

9. John Abel to Mary Hinman, 11 March, 1 April 1883, Abel Papers, record group 1. On Vaughan, see Horace W. Davenport, *Physiology, 1850–1923: The View from Michigan*, supplement to *Physiologist* 24, no. 1, (February 1982): 17–19, and Leigh C. Anderson, "Victor Clarence Vaughan," in Wyndham D. Miles, ed., *American Chemists and Chemical Engineers* (Washington, D.C.: American Chemical Society, 1976), pp. 484–85.

10. John Abel to Mary Hinman, 26 November 1882, 18 February and 25 March 1883, Abel Papers, record group 1.

11. On Sewall, see Davenport, *Physiology*, 25–38.

12. John Abel to Mary Hinman, 14 April 1883, Abel Papers, record group 1.

13. John Abel to Mary Hinman, 25 February 1883, Abel Papers, record group 1.

14. John Abel to Mary Hinman, 1 April 1883, Abel Papers, record group 1.

15. Mary Abel to Kate Daniels, 15 February 1884, Abel Papers, record group 1; transcribed copy of letter from John Abel to Mary Hinman, 16 June 1880, Abel Papers, record group 8 (see the reference to the Geiling Materials in footnote 1 to this chapter; the original letter appears to have been lost).

16. Mary Abel to Ella Swift, 6 February 1884, Abel Papers, record group 1.

17. Thomas Bonner, *American Doctors and German Universities: A Chapter in International Relations, 1870–1914* (Lincoln: University of Nebraska Press, 1963), pp. 13–14. See also Robert G. Frank, Jr., "American Physiologists in German Laboratories, 1865–1914," in Gerald L. Geison, ed., *Physiology in the American Context* (Bethesda, Md.: American Physiological Society, 1987), pp. 11–46.

18. John Abel to Mary Abel, 1 and 5 June 1884, Abel Papers, record group 1.

19. John Abel to Mary Abel, 5 and 8 June 1884, Abel Papers, record group 1.

20. John Abel to Mary Abel, 20 and 22 June 1884, Abel Papers, record group 1.

21. Mary Abel to Kate Daniels, 27 July 1884, Abel Papers, record group 1.

22. Mary Abel to unknown person [probably her friend Ella Swift], 12 May 1884 [incomplete handwritten letter, headed "Life Plans—Going to Germany"], Abel Papers, record group 1.

23. See Robert E. Kohler, *From Medical Chemistry to Biochemistry: The Making of a Biomedical Discipline* (Cambridge: Cambridge University Press, 1982), pp. 121–57 and Kenneth M. Ludmerer, *Learning to Heal: The Development of American Medical Education* (New York: Basic Books, 1985), pp. 29–138.

24. Ludmerer, *Learning to Heal*, p. 47.

25. On American students working in Ludwig's laboratory, see George Rosen, "Carl Ludwig and His American Students," *Bull. Hist. Med.* 4 (1936): 609–50 and Frank, "American Physiologists," pp. 32–37.

26. Mary Abel to Kate Daniels, 22 October 1884, Abel Papers, record group 1.

27. Drafts of letters from John Abel to Horatio Wood, 24 June 1888 and to G. Stanley Hall, June 1888, Abel Papers, record group 1.

28. Frank, "American Physiologists," p. 28. I am using the term *German* here, as is generally done with respect to this subject, to include Austrian, Swiss, and other universities of Germanic language and tradition.

29. Mary Abel to Ella Swift, 5 June 1886, Abel Papers, record group 1. The decision to stay longer in Germany had been made well before that time, however. Earlier that year, Mary wrote that they would be in Germany two years more and probably longer. Mary Abel to Mrs. Talbot, 23 February 1886, Abel Papers, record group 1.

30. Copy of letter from Frank Schaefer to E. M. K. Geiling, 13 February 1958, Abel Papers, record group 8; Mary Abel to Ella Swift, 5 June 1886 and notes from John Abel concerning money borrowed from his father against John's share of family property, 24 June 1889, 8 July 1890, and undated, Abel Papers, record group 1.

31. Kohler, *Medical Chemistry*, p. 23.

32. John Abel to Frances Hinman, 27 March 1885; Mary Abel to Kate Daniels, 8 January 1886; copy of letter from John Abel to G. Stanley Hall, June 1888; copy of letter from Abel to Horatio Wood, 24 June 1888; Abel Papers, record group 1.

33. Copy of letter from John Abel to Horatio Wood, 24 June 1888, Abel Papers, record group 1.

34. Ibid.; E. M. K. Geiling, "John J. Abel and Family, U.S. and Europe," 5-page undated typescript, Abel Papers, record group 8.

35. Copy of letter from John Abel to Henry Sewall, June 1888, Abel Papers, record group 1. See also copies of letters from Abel to H. N. Martin, June 1888; to William Welch, 18 June 1888; to G. S. Hall, June 1888; to Horatio Wood, 24 June 1888; Abel Papers, record group 1.

36. Copy of letter from John Abel to Horatio Wood, 24 June 1888, Abel Papers, record group 1.

37. Mary Abel to Katherine Daniels, 26 May 1889, Abel Papers, record group 1. See also Frances Hinman to person unknown, 8 January 1889, ibid. and Geiling, "John J. Abel and Family."

38. Frances Hinman to person unknown, 8 January 1889, Abel Papers, record group 1.

39. Mary Hinman Abel, *Practical Sanitary and Economic Cooking Adapted to Persons of Moderate and Small Means: The Lomb Prize Essay* (n.p.: American Public Health Association, 1890). See also Mary Abel to her sister Estelle, 8 August 1888 and Frances Hinman to person unknown, 8 January 1888, Abel Papers, record group 1.

40. John Abel to Mary Abel, 18 September 1889, Abel Papers, record group 1.

41. Mary Abel to her sister Estelle (with handwritten note added by Frances Hinman), March 1889 and John Abel to Mary Abel, 22 September 1889, Abel Papers, record group 1.

42. John Abel to Mary Abel, 22 September, 1 and 27 October 1889, Abel Papers, record group 1.

43. John Abel to Mary Abel, 27 and 31 October 1889, 6 April 1890 and John Abel to Frances Hinman, 15 April 1890, Abel Papers, record group 1.

44. Geiling, "John J. Abel and Family" and Janet Wilson James, "Ellen Henrietta Swallow Richards," in Edward T. James, Janet Wilson James, and Paul S. Boyer, eds., *Notable American Women, 1607–1950: A Biographical Dictionary* (Cambridge: Harvard University Press, 1971), 3: 143–46.

45. Mary Abel to Frances Hinman, 16 November 1889, Abel Papers, record group 1; James, "Ellen Henrietta Swallow Richards," p. 145; [Mary Abel], *The Story of the New England Kitchen* (Boston: 1890); "Mary Hinman Abel—1850–1938," *J. Home Econ.* 30 (1938): 361.

46. Mary Abel to John Abel, 2 and 4 February, 21 April 1890 and John Abel to Mary Abel, 18 May 1890, Abel Papers, record group 1. On women studying in Swiss medical schools, see Thomas Bonner, "Medical Women Abroad: A New Dimension of Women's Push for Opportunity in Medicine, 1850–1914," *Bull. Hist. Med.* 62 (1988): 58–73.

47. Mary Abel to John Abel, 4 February, 13 April, 22 May 1890, Abel Papers, record group 1.

48. Mary Abel to John Abel, 22 May, 21 June 1890 and John Abel to Mary Abel, 22 March 1890, Abel papers, record group 1.

49. Kate Farrand Reighard to Mary Abel, 28 May 1890; Mary Abel to John Abel, 31 May 1890; Mary Abel to Frances Hinman, 1 June 1890; copy of letter from Mary Abel to Victor Vaughan, undated; copy of letter from John Abel to Victor Vaughan, 1 June 1890; John Abel to Mary Abel, 1 June 1890; Abel Papers, record group 1.

50. John Abel to Mary Abel, 22 and 29 June, 4 July 1890; Mary Abel to Frances Hinman, 21 July 1890; copy of letter from John Abel to Victor Vaughan, undated; Abel Papers, record group 1.

51. John Abel to Mary Abel, 6 June 1890, Abel Papers, record group 1.

52. Copy of letter from John Abel to Victor Vaughan, 15 July 1890, Abel Papers, record group 1.

53. Victor Vaughan to John Abel, 1 July 1890, Abel Papers, record group 1.

54. Frederick G. Novy, "The Administration and Curriculum" (medical school), in Wilfred B. Shaw, ed., Part V of *The University of Michigan: An Encyclopedic Survey* (Ann Arbor: University of Michigan Press, 1941–58), pp. 773–808 (the quotation is from p. 805).

55. Ibid., pp. 804–6.

56. Henry H. Swain, E. M. K. Geiling, and Alexander Heingartner, "John Jacob Abel at Michigan: The Introduction of Pharmacology into the Medical Curriculum," *Univ. Michigan Med. Bull.* 29 (1963): 1–14, especially pp. 5–6.

Chapter Three   Abel and the Beginnings of Pharmacology
in American Medical Schools

1. Copy of letter from John Abel to Victor Vaughan, 15 July 1890; John Abel to Mary Abel, 4 August 1890; Abel Papers, record group 1.

2. John Abel to Mary Abel, 25 July 1890, Abel Papers, record group 1.

3. John Abel to Mary Abel, 24 July 1890, Abel Papers, record group 1.

4. John Abel to C. W. Edmunds, 24 May 1937. The original letter is in the Department of Pharmacology at the University of Michigan, Ann Arbor. A copy is in the Abel Papers, record group 1.

5. Copy of letter from John Abel to Victor Vaughan, 15 July 1890; John Abel to Mary Abel, 21 July 1890; Abel Papers, record group 1.

6. Abel to Edmunds, 24 May 1937 and Edmund Drechsel to John Abel, 2 October 1890, Abel Papers, record group 1.

7. John Abel to Mary Abel, 21 July 1890; Victor Vaughan to John Abel, 1 August 1890; James Angell to John Abel, 15 September 1890; Abel Papers, record group 1.

8. Victor C. Vaughan, *A Doctor's Memories* (Indianapolis: Bobbs-Merrill, 1926), p. 216. An account of Abel's tenure at Michigan cites this statement of Vaughan's as evidence that he "saw and seized the opportunity to make the change from classical materia medica to modern pharmacology" when the chair of materia medica was vacated by the firing of Frothingham (chapter 2). See Henry H. Swain, E. M. K. Geiling, and Alexander Heingartner, "John Jacob Abel at Michigan: The Introduction of Pharmacology into the Medical Curriculum" *Univ. Michigan Med. Bull.* 29 (1963): 1–14 (the quotation is from p. 6).

9. For example, Vaughan did not mention in his correspondence with Abel about the appointment (cited above) that he wished to convert the position from materia medica to pharmacology nor that he had been in touch with Schmiedeberg. Nor did Schmiedeberg mention any previous contact with Vaughan when he wrote to Abel informing him that he had complied with his request to write a letter of reference of his behalf (Oswald Schmiedeberg to John Abel, 21 July 1890, Abel Papers, record group 1).

10. Victor Vaughan to John Abel, 1 August 1890, Abel Papers, record group 1. Vaughan was not actually appointed as dean of the medical school until 1891, but he apparently played some role in the selection of faculty (such as Abel) even before that time. In his autobiography he claimed that when Ford became dean in 1887, he "practically turned over that function to me" (Vaughan, *Memories*, p. 213). Vaughan may have been exaggerating his authority here, however, as we have already seen that his recollections were not always accurate.

11. Abel to Edmunds, 24 May 1937 (see note 4).

12. Ibid.

13. This discussion of Abel's work at Michigan is based largely on Abel's recollections in his previously cited letter to Edmunds, 24 May 1937, as well as on information in the *Calendar of the University of Michigan* and the "Proceedings of the Board of Regents, University of Michigan," Michigan Historical Collections, Bentley Historical Library, University of Michigan, Ann Arbor, for the period 1891–93. Other sources of useful information on Abel and pharmacology at Michigan are Swain, Geiling, and Heingartner,

"John Jacob Abel at Michigan"; Charles W. Edmunds, "The Department of Materia Medica and Therapeutics," in Wilfred B. Shaw, ed., Part V of *The University of Michigan: An Encycopedic Survey* (Ann Arbor: University of Michigan Press, 1941–58), pp. 845–55; Horace W. Davenport, *Fifty Years of Medicine at the University of Michigan, 1891–1941* (Ann Arbor: University of Michigan Medical School, 1986), pp. 111–34.

14. John J. Abel, "The Methods of Pharmacology, with Experimental Illustrations," *Pharm. Era* 7 (1892): 105–7 (the quotation is from p. 105).

15. Ibid., pp. 105–6.

16. John J. Abel and Archibald Muirhead, "Ueber das Vorkommen der Carbaminsäure im Menschen- und Hundeharn nach reichlichem Genuss von Kalkhydrat," *Arch. Exp. Pathol. Pharmakol.* 31 (1892): 15–29; John J. Abel, "Ueber das Vorkommen von Aethylsulfid in Hundeharn, über das Verhalten seiner Lösung in concentrirter Schwefelsäure gegen Oxydationsmittel und über einige Reactionen zur Auffindung der Alkylsulfide," *Z. Physiol. Chem.* 20 (1894): 253–79.

17. John Abel to Mary Abel, 17 July 1892, Abel Papers, record group 1.

18. John Abel to Mary Abel, 8 June 1892, Abel Papers, record group 1.

19. Abel to Edmunds, 24 May 1937.

20. John Abel to Mary Abel, 25 and 29 September 1892, Abel Papers, record group 1.

21. Alan Mason Chesney, *The Johns Hopkins Hospital and the Johns Hopkins University School of Medicine: A Chronicle* (Baltimore: Johns Hopkins Press, 1943–58), 1: 95–97; A. McGehee Harvey, et al., *A Model of Its Kind. A Centennial History of Medicine at Johns Hopkins* (Baltimore: Johns Hopkins University Press, 1989), 1: 27–28, 137–41.

22. Medical Faculty Advisory Board Minutes, 12 January 1893, 1: 26, Alan Mason Chesney Medical Archives, The Johns Hopkins Medical Institutions, Baltimore; William Osler to John Abel, 13 January 1893, Abel Papers, record group 1.

23. D. C. Gilman to John Abel, 5 July 1882; Ira Remsen to John Abel, 28 May 1884; Copy of letter from John Abel to D.C. Gilman, 18 June 1888; copy of letter from John Abel to H. N. Martin, June 1888; copy of letter from John Abel to William Welch, 18 June 1888; Abel Papers, record group 1.

24. Copy of letter from John Abel to William Welch, 18 June 1888; William Welch to John Abel, 14 May 1892; John Abel to Mary Abel, June 1892; William Osler to John Abel, 26 March 1892; Abel Papers, record group 1.

25. William Osler to John Abel, 2 March 1893 and copy of letter from John Abel to William Osler, 7 March 1893, Abel Papers, record group 1; Medical Faculty Advisory Board Minutes, 2 March 1893, 1: 40, Chesney Archives; John Abel to William Osler, 16 March 1893, Daniel Coit Gilman Papers, John Jacob Abel correspondence, Special Collections, Eisenhower

Library, Johns Hopkins University, Baltimore. In his original letter to Abel in January, cited earlier, Osler had also spoken of pharmacology rather than materia medica.

26. John Abel to W. L. Biering, 18 February 1924, Abel Papers, record group 1. Silas H. Douglass, for example, had the title of professor of chemistry, pharmacology, and materia medica at the University of Michigan in 1850. See David Cowen, "Materia Medica and Pharmacology," in Ronald Numbers, ed., *The Education of American Physicians: Historical Essays* (Berkeley: University of California Press, 1980), pp. 95–121, see p. 99.

27. Chesney, *Johns Hopkins*, 1: 227–28, 2: 95–100.

28. John Abel to William Osler, 3 April 1893 and John Abel to Daniel Gilman, 2 and 16 April 1893, Gilman Papers, Abel correspondence. Daniel Gilman to John Abel, 13 April 1893 and William Welch to John Abel, 19 and 20 April 1893, Abel Papers, record group 1.

29. William Welch to John Abel, 20 April 1893, Abel Papers, record group 1.

30. Arthur Cushny to John Abel, 25 June 1893; John Abel to Walter Dixon, 18 March 1926; John Abel to A. J. Clark, 9 April 1926; Abel Papers, record group 1. "Proceedings of the Board of Regents, University of Michigan, 1891–96," Bentley Library, "Special Meeting, August, 1893" (3 August 1893). Swain, Geiling and Heingartner, "Abel at Michigan," p. 14. Vaughan (*Doctor's Memories*, p. 216) claimed that he wrote to Schmiedeberg, who recommended Cushny, when Abel resigned. As we have seen, however, Vaughan's memory was faulty in recounting the story of Abel's appointment. In the case of Cushny, the evidence suggests that Abel played a major part in bringing him to Michigan.

31. On Cushny, see the biography by Gerald Geison in *Dictionary of Scientific Biography* (New York: Charles Scribner's Sons, 1978), 15: 99–104; John Abel, "Arthur Robertson Cushny and Pharmacology," *J. Pharmacol. Exp. Ther.* 27 (1926): 265–86; Helen MacGillivray, "A Personal Biography of Arthur Robertson Cushny, 1866–1926," *Annu. Rev. Pharmacol.* 8 (1968): 1–24.

32. Edmunds, "Materia Medica," p. 349; Davenport, "Fifty Years of Medicine," pp. 122–23; Charles Edmunds and Arthur Cushny, *Laboratory Guide in Experimental Pharmacology* (Ann Arbor, Mich.: George Wahr, 1905).

33. Edmunds and Cushny, *Laboratory Guide*, p. 95.

34. Ibid., p. 203.

35. John J. Abel, "On the Teaching of Pharmacology, Materia Medica, and Therapeutics in Our Medical Schools," *Philadelphia Med. J.* 6 (1900): 384–90 (the quotation is from p. 387). This article was reprinted in *John Jacob Abel, M.D., Investigator, Teacher, Prophet, 1857–1938: A Collection of Papers by and about the Father of American Pharmacology* (Baltimore: Williams and Wilkins, 1957), pp. 57–72.

36. See Merriley Borrell, "Instruments and an Independent Physiology:

The Harvard Physiological Laboratory, 1871–1906," in Geison, *Physiology in the American Context*, pp. 293–321.

37. John Abel to Torald Sollman, January 1909 and John Abel to Albert Crawford, 3 March 1920, Abel Papers, record group 1; Paul Lamson, "John Jacob Abel: A Portrait," *Bull. Johns Hopkins Hosp.* 68 (1941): 119–57, see p. 146. The Lamson article was reprinted in *John Jacob Abel, M.D.*, pp. 8–42.

38. Lamson, "John Jacob Abel," pp. 145–46.

39. Ibid., pp. 146–147.

40. See the recollections of Abel's associates about his laboratory, such as ibid.; Leonard Rowntree, "John Jacob Abel, Decade, 1903–1913," *Bull. Johns Hopkins Hosp.* 101 (1957): 306–10; E. K. Marshall, Jr., "John Jacob Abel, Decade, 1913–1923," ibid., 311–16; E. M. K. Geiling, "John Jacob Abel, Decade, 1923–1932," ibid., 317–26.

41. For Abel's views on the training of pharmacologists, see John Abel to Abraham Flexner, 12 March 1920 and 5 June 1922; John Abel to Charles Erlanger, 20 January 1921; John Abel to M. M. Zinninger, 14 October 1929; John Abel to George Roth, 28 November 1930; Abel Papers, record group 1. The date for the beginning of a formal Ph.D. program in pharmacology at Johns Hopkins is taken from Elliot S. Vesell, ed., *Survey of Pharmacology in Medical Schools of North America* (Nutley, N.J.: Association for Medical School Pharmacology and American Society for Pharmacology and Experimental Therapeutics, 1974), p. 134.

42. Lamson, "John Jacob Abel," p. 154. Others have also commented on how Abel provided little in the way of detailed direction for their research, e.g., Marshall, "John Jacob Abel," p. 314.

43. Marshall, "John Jacob Abel," p. 314.

44. Geiling, "John Jacob Abel," p. 319.

45. John Abel to Mrs. Franklin, 13 October 1920, Abel Papers, record group 1; "Dr. Abel at Work in Laboratory Two Days After Leg is Broken," *Baltimore Sun*, 13 January 1926; "Hopkins Professor Injured" [1900], "The Chemicals Explode" [1900], "Dangerous Drug Explodes" (dated by hand 21 March 1902), unidentified newspaper clippings, Abel Papers, record group 7.

46. See the previously cited recollections by his associates.

47. Ibid.

48. Rowntree, "John Jacob Abel," p. 307.

49. Carl Voegtlin, "John Jacob Abel, 1857–1938," *J. Pharmacol. Exp. Ther.* 67 (1939): 373–406, especially pp. 377–78.

50. On the history of epinephrine or adrenaline, see Horace W. Davenport, "Epinephrin(e)," *Physiologist* 25 (1982): 76–82.

51. John J. Abel and Albert C. Crawford, "On the Blood-Pressure-Raising Constituent of the Suprarenal Capsule," *Bull. Johns Hopkins Hosp.* 8 (1897): 151–57.

52. John J. Abel, "Further Observations on the Chemical Nature of the

Active Principle of the Suprarenal Capsule," *Bull. Johns Hopkins Hosp.* 9 (1898): 215–18; John J. Abel, "Ueber den blutdruckerregenden Bestandtheil des Nebenniere, das Epinephrin," *Hoppe-Seyler's Z. Physiol. Chem.* 28 (1899): 318–62.

53. Jokichi Takamine, "The Blood-Pressure-Raising Principle of the Suprarenal Glands—A Preliminary Report," *Ther. Gaz.* 17 (1901): 221–24; Jokichi Takamine, "Adrenalin the Active Principle of the Suprarenal Glands and Its Mode of Preparation," *Am. J. Pharm.* 73 (1901): 523–31.

54. T. B. Aldrich, "A Preliminary Report on the Active Principle of the Suprarenal Gland," *Am. J. Physiol.* 5 (1901): 457–61.

55. For a discussion of the controversy, see Davenport, "Epinephrin(e)," pp. 80–81.

56. John J. Abel and L. G. Rowntree, "On the Pharmacological Action of Some Phthaleins and Their Derivatives, with Especial Reference to Their Behavior as Purgatives. I.," *J. Pharmacol. Exp. Ther.* 1 (1909): 231–64. The quotation on the condition of the stools is from p. 246.

57. On Abel's research on vividiffusion, pituitary extract, and the other topics mentioned, see Voegtlin, "John Jacob Abel," and William deB. MacNider, "John Jacob Abel, 1857–1938," *Biog. Mem. Natl. Acad. Sci.* 24 (1947): 231–57, both of which contain bibliographies of Abel's publications. On the early development of an artificial kidney for clinical use, see Jost Benedum, "Georg Haas (1886–1971), Pionier der Hämodialyse," *Medizinhist. J.* 14 (1979): 196–217; Willem J. Kolff, "First Clinical Experience with the Artificial Kidney," *Ann. Intern. Med.* 62 (1965): 608–19.

58. The discussion of Abel's insulin research is based largely upon Jane H. Murnaghan and Paul Talalay, "John Jacob Abel and the Crystallization of Insulin," *Perspect. Biol. Med.* 10 (1967): 334–80.

59. John J. Abel, "Crystalline Insulin," *Proc. Natl. Acad. Sci. USA* 12 (1926): 132–36.

60. For a discussion of Abel's difficulties in repeating his original success and of the controversy over the adsorption theory, see Murnaghan and Talalay, "John Jacob Abel," pp. 346–68.

61. Ibid, pp. 368–76.

Chapter Four   The Growth of Academic Pharmacology in the United States

1. Kenneth M. Ludmerer, *Learning to Heal: The Development of American Medical Education* (New York: Basic Books, 1985); William G. Rothstein, *American Medical Schools and the Practice of Medicine: A History* (New York: Oxford University Press, 1987).

2. Ludmerer, *Learning to Heal*, pp. 43–101.

3. Rothstein, *American Medical Schools*, p. 106.

4. Ludmerer, *Learning to Heal*, p. 83.

5. For a bibliography on the history of academic pharmacology in the United States, see John Parascandola and Elizabeth Keeney, *Sources in the History of American Pharmacology* (Madison, Wis.: American Institute of the History of Pharmacy, 1983), pp. 11–18. For a useful overview, including extensive references, see David Cowen, "Materia Medica and Pharmacology," in Ronald L. Numbers, ed., *The Education of American Physicians: Historical Essays* (Berkeley: University of California Press, 1980), pp. 95–121.

6. Robert E. Kohler, *From Medical Chemistry to Biochemistry: The Making of a Biomedical Discipline* (Cambridge: Cambridge University Press, 1982), pp. 158–68.

7. Quoted from ibid., pp. 159–60. The statement is from a letter of 20 August 1980 from Alsberg to Charles W. Eliot in the Eliot Papers at the Harvard University Archives.

8. Frederick C. Waite, *Western Reserve University Centennial History of the School of Medicine* (Cleveland: Western Reserve University Press, 1946), pp. 347, 525, 563; Torald Sollmann, "Why an Annual Review of Pharmacology?" *Annu. Rev. Pharmacol.* 1 (1961): 1–6, p. 5.

9. *The Medical College of Western Reserve University, Announcement*, 1895–96, pp. 8, 15–16 (the quotation is from p. 16).

10. Waite, *Western Reserve*, p. 347; Sollmann, "Annual Review," pp. 4–5; *The Medical College of Western Reserve, Announcement*, 1896–97, 1897–98, 1898–99, 1899–1900.

11. See G. P. Jenkins, "Sollmann, Torald Hermann," in Martin Kaufman, Stuart Galishoff, and Todd Savitt, eds., *Dictionary of American Medical Biography* (Westport, Conn.: Greenwood Press, 1984), 2: 705; "T. H. Sollmann—Pharmacologist," *Postgrad. Med.* 1 (1947): 328–32, p. 329.

12. On Sollmann's career, see Sollmann, "Annual Review"; "T. H. Sollmann—Pharmacologist"; Parascandola and Keeney, *Sources*, pp. 50–51.

13. Torald Sollmann, *A Textbook of Pharmacology and Some Allied Sciences* (Philadelphia: W. B. Saunders, 1901); Torald Sollmann, *A Manual of Pharmacology and Its Applications to Therapeutics and Toxicology* (Philadelphia: W. B. Saunders, 1917).

14. On Hatcher, see Parascandola and Keeney, *Sources*, pp. 35–36; Harry Gold, "Hatcher, Robert Anthony," in *Dictionary of American Biography* (New York: Charles Scribner's Sons, 1973), suppl. 3, pp. 342–43. On Wallace, see Parascandola and Keeney, *Sources*, pp. 57–58; the obituary by William deBerniere MacNider, "George Barclay Wallace, 1874–1948," *J. Pharmacol. Exp. Ther.* 93 (1948): 127–28. Hatcher was appointed as an instructor in pharmacology at Cornell in 1904 and promoted to professor four years later. Wallace was appointed as an instructor in pharmacology at New York University and became a professor there in 1907.

15. On Herter, see Robert M. Hawthorne, Jr., "Christian Archibald Herter, M.D. (1865–1910)," *Perspect. Biol. Med.* 18 (1974): 24–39.

16. F. S. Lee, "The School of Medicine (College of Physicians and Sur-

geons)," in *A History of Columbia University, 1754–1904* (New York: Columbia University Press, 1904), pp. 307–34 (the quotation is from pp. 330–31).

17. Carl F. Schmidt, "Alfred Newton Richards 1876–1966," *Ann. Intern. Med.* suppl. 8 (1969): 15–27, p. 17; Carl F. Schmidt, "Alfred Newton Richards 1876–1966," *Biog. Mem. Fellows R. Soc.* 13 (1967): 327–42, p. 329.

18. Kohler, *Biochemistry*, p. 115.

19. Leslie B. Arey, *Northwestern University Medical School, 1859–1979: A Pioneer in Educational Reform* (Evanston, Ill.: Northwestern University, 1979), p. 171; *Northwestern University Medical School Circular of Information*, published annually, for the 1890s.

20. J. H. Long to Abel, 23 October 1907, Abel Papers; *Northwestern University Medical School Circular of Information*, 1906–7, 1908–9. The dean of the medical school wrote to Abel in 1909 to thank him for recommending Richards, with whom they were very satisfied; Arthur Edwards to Abel, 1 February 1909, Abel Papers.

21. Paul F. Clark, *The University of Wisconsin Medical School, A Chronicle, 1848–1948* (Madison: University of Wisconsin Press, 1967), pp. 3–21.

22. On the Wisconsin pharmacology program, see ibid., pp. 95–104. For biographical information on Loevenhart, see Parascandola and Keeney, *Sources*, pp. 40–42.

23. James W. Fisher and Kathleen Carter, "History of Pharmacology at Tulane," *Tulane Med.* 1 (1969): 4, 6, 14.

24. Chalmers Gemmill and Mary Jeanne Jones, *Pharmacology at the University of Virginia School of Medicine* (Charlottesville: University of Virginia Department of Pharmacology, 1966), pp. 99–107.

25. John J. Abel, "Albert Cornelius Crawford," *J. Pharmacol. Exp. Ther.* 18 (1921): 5; Albert Crawford to John Abel, 12 November 1910, Abel Papers.

26. David Starr Jordan to John Abel, 30 October 1909, 8 April 1910 and C. W. Edmunds to John Abel, 21 and 26 March, 17 April 1910, Abel Papers.

27. David Starr Jordan to John Abel, 30 October 1909, Abel Papers.

28. Abraham Flexner, *Medical Education in the United States and Canada: A Report to the Carnegie Foundation for the Advancement of Teaching* (New York: The Carnegie Foundation for the Advancement of Teaching, 1910), pp. 28, 71–89.

29. Flexner, *Medical Education*, pp. 63–65.

30. *Catalogue of the University of Pennsylvania*, 1896–97, pp. 226–30, 240–43 (the quotation is from p. 242).

31. Medical Faculty Minutes, University of Pennsylvania, 15 November 1897, 17 January and 21 February 1898, University of Pennsylvania Archives, Philadelphia.

32. *Catalogue of the University of Pennsylvania*, 1898–99, pp. 238, 250; ibid., 1903–4, pp. 299–301; Medical Faculty Minutes, University of Pennsylvania, 16 November 1903.

33. Board of Trustees Minutes, University of Pennsylvania, 7 March 1905, University of Pennsylvania Archives, Philadelphia; letter from Horatio C Wood to John Abel, 1 March 1905, Abel Papers.

34. Medical Faculty Minutes, University of Pennsylvania, 17 December 1906.

35. George W. Corner, *Two Centuries of Medicine: A History of the School of Medicine, University of Pennsylvania* (Philadelphia: J. B. Lippincott Co., 1965), pp. 210–18.

36. Arthur Cushny to John Abel, 31 December 1907, Abel Papers.

37. Corner, *Two Centuries*, p. 217; *Catalogue of the University of Pennsylvania*, 1907–8, pp. 393–95.

38. Undated copy of letter from David Edsall to Torald Sollmann written in connection with work of a Committee on Pharmacology, Toxicology, and Therapeutics of the American Medical Association's Council on Medical Education (established in 1908 to study the medical curriculum), in Circular 4 from Sollmann to the members of the committee, 28 November 1908, Abel Papers.

39. On H. C. Wood, Jr., see J. McKeen Cattell and Jacques Cattell, *American Men of Science: A Biographical Directory*, 5th ed. (New York: Science Press, 1933), p. 1231. On Edsall, see Joseph C. Aub and Ruth K. Hapgood, *Pioneer in Modern Medicine: David Linn Edsall of Harvard* (n.p.: Harvard Medical Alumni Association, 1970).

40. Board of Trustees Minutes, University of Pennsylvania, 17 May, 7 June 1910; *Catalogue of the University of Pennsylvania*, 1910–11, pp. 439–440, 443.

41. On Richards, see Schmidt, "Richards," *Ann Intern. Med.* and Schmidt, "Richards," *Biog. Mem. Fellows R. Soc.*

42. Corner, *Two Centuries*, pp. 250–52.

43. *The Harvard Medical School, 1782–1906* (n.p., 1906), pp. 163–69 (the quotation is from p. 163).

44. *Annual Catalogue of the Medical School of Harvard University*, 1871–72, p. 4. See also *Harvard Medical School*, pp. 165–66.

45. Henry K. Beecher and Mark D. Altschule, *Medicine at Harvard: The First Three Hundred Years* (Hanover, N.H.: University Press of New England, 1977), pp. 87–101.

46. *Catalogue of the Medical School of Harvard*, 1884–85, pp. 174–75, 185, 192. In the narrative discussion of the curriculum, there is a reference (p. 185) to a course of lectures on "experimental pharmacology," but the course title and the title of the instructor both refer to "experimental therapeutics." Ibid., 1885–86, pp. 188, 198–99, 205. See also editions of the *Catalogue* over the next few years.

47. For biographical information on Williams, see Otto Glaser, "Williams, Francis Henry," in *Dictionary of American Biography* (New York: Charles Scribner's Sons, 1958), suppl. 2, pp. 717–18. On Williams and

Schmiedeberg, see John Abel to Mary Abel, 22 March and 8 June 1890 and Mary Abel to John Abel, 22 May 1890, Abel Papers.

48. *Catalogue of the Medical School of Harvard* 1895–96, pp. 199, 205; Mary Abel to John Abel, 22 May 1890, Abel Papers.

49. *Catalogue of the Medical School of Harvard*, 1895–96, pp. 9, 34, 41 (the quotation is from p. 34).

50. Very little biographical information is available on Pfaff. See the brief biographical sketches in Allen G. Debus, ed., *World Who's Who in Science* (Chicago: Marquis–Who's Who, 1968), p. 1339; J. McKeen Cattell, *American Men of Science* (New York: Science Press, 1906), p. 251.

51. *Harvard University Catalogue*, 1903–4, p. 621; letter from Franz Pfaff to John Abel, 7 March 1910, Abel Papers.

52. For citations to Pfaff's publication through 1900, see Royal Society of London, *Catalogue of Scientific Papers, Fourth Series (1884–1900)* (Cambridge: Cambridge University Press, 1921), 17: 836.

53. Arthur Loevenhart to John Abel, 7 January 1909 and Torald Sollmann to John Abel, 18 January 1909, Abel Papers.

54. Franz Pfaff to John Abel, 7 March 1910, Abel Papers; Walter Cannon to Edward Bradford, 17 May 1912, Dean's Office Subject Files, Harvard Medical School, Countway Library, Boston.

55. See the entry prepared by the department itself in Elliot S. Vesell, ed., *Survey of Pharmacology in Medical Schools of North America* (Nutley, N.J.: Association for Medical School Pharmacology and American Society for Pharmacology and Experimental Therapeutics, 1974), p. 104.

56. For biographical information on Hunt, see E. K. Marshall, Jr., "Reid Hunt, 1870–1948," *Biog. Mem. Natl. Acad. Sci.* 26 (1951): 25–44; Parascandola and Keeney, *Sources*, pp. 38–40.

57. Isaac Hall Manning and Walter Reece Berryhill, "Medical Education at the University of North Carolina," in Dorothy Long, ed., *Medicine in North Carolina: Essays in the History of Medical Science and Medical Service, 1524–1960* (Raleigh: North Carolina Medical Society, 1972), 2: 373–483, especially pp. 376–81.

58. *University of North Carolina, The Medical School*, 1900, pp. 7–8.

59. Manning and Berryhill, "Medical Education," pp. 383–88; *The University of North Carolina Catalogue*, 1903–4, p. 77 and 1904–5, p. 84. For biographical information on MacNider, see A. N. Richards, "William deBerniere MacNider, June 25, 1881–May 31, 1951," *Biog. Mem. Natl. Acad. Sci.* 32 (1958): 238–272; William deBerniere MacNider, *The Good Doctor and Other Selections from Essays and Addresses* (Chapel Hill, N.C.: University of North Carolina, 1953).

60. Manning and Berryhill, "Medical Education," pp. 387–88. Venable was concerned enough about the situation that he wrote to several individuals to assure them that the university had no intention of allowing the Department of Medicine to be weakened after the resignation of Whitehead. See the letter

from Venable to V. A. Ward, 13 August 1905, box 21, folder 784, University of North Carolina Records, University Archives, Manuscripts Department, University of North Carolina Library, Chapel Hill.

61. Francis Venable to Richard Whitehead, 19, 24, and 29 July 1905 and R. H. Lewis to Francis Venable, 20 and 29 July 1905, University of North Carolina Records, box 21, folders 782–83.

62. R. H. Lewis to Francis Venable, 29 July 1905, University of North Carolina Records, box 21, folder 783.

63. Francis Venable to R. H. Lewis, 1 August 1905 and Francis Venable to William MacNider, 31 July 1905, University of North Carolina Records, box 21, folders 783–84; Manning and Berryhill, "Medical Education," pp. 387–88. See also the catalogues of the medical school for this period.

64. Report of the Dean of the Medical School at Chapel Hill, 1905, University of North Carolina Trustee Minutes, vol. S–11, p. 79, University Archives, North Carolina Library, Chapel Hill; *The University of North Carolina Catalogue*, 1905–6, pp. 91, 94, 100–101; *The University of North Carolina Record Describing the Departments of Medicine and Pharmacy*, no. 28, April 1904, pp. 9–10, no. 42, February 1906, pp. 12–13, no. 50, February 1907, p. 13.

65. Manning and Berryhill, "Medical Education," p. 388; Fred W. Ellis, "A History of Pharmacology at the University of North Carolina at Chapel Hill," *North Carolina Med. J.* 40 (1979): 555–59, p. 556; Report of the Dean of the Medical School at Chapel Hill, 1906, University of North Carolina Trustee Minutes, vol. S–11, p. 130.

66. William deBerniere MacNider, "The Teaching of Pharmacology in the Smaller Medical Schools," *Southern Med. J.* 2 (1909): 904–7 (the quotation is from p. 907).

67. *Graduate Training in Pharmacology Programs in the United States and Canada* (Bethesda, Md: American Society for Pharmacology and Experimental Therapeutics, 1988). For some information on pharmacology in other health professions schools, see M. L. Tainter, "The Place of Pharmacology in Dental Education and Methods of Instruction," *J. Dent. Educ.* 2 (1938): 212–23; Debra P. Hymovich and Marjorie P. Jones, "Whither Pharmacology in the Curriculum," *Nurs. Outlook* 16, no. 8 (1968): 58–60; Lloyd E. Davis, "Pharmacology Training in Schools of Veterinary Medicine," *Fed. Proc.* 36 (1975): 119–23.

68. Robert L. Talbert and Charles A. Walton, "An Integrated Approach to Instruction in Pharmacology and Therapeutics," *Am. J. Pharm. Educ.* 40 (1976): 369–77 (the quotation is from p. 369); Linwood Tice, "Pharmacy Education for Today and the Future," (unpublished paper presented at the Medical College of South Carolina, 28 October 1966, pp. 6–7; copy in Kremers Reference Files, C31aI, F. B. Power Pharmaceutical Library, University of Wisconsin–Madison).

69. The discussion that follows is based on John Parascandola and John

Swann, "Development of Pharmacology in American Schools of Pharmacy," *Pharm. Hist.* 25 (1983): 95–115.

70. Ibid., pp. 97–99.

71. Ibid., pp. 100–101. See the *Annual Announcement of the School of Pharmacy of the University of Michigan* for the 1880s and 1890s. See also Henry Swain, E. M. K. Geiling, and Alexander Heingartner, "John Jacob Abel at Michigan: The Introduction of Pharmacology into the Medical Curriculum," *Univ. Michigan Med. Bull.* 19 (1963): 1–14, p. 10.

72. Parascandola and Swann, "Pharmacology," pp. 101–2. See also Jennie Tom, "Rufus Ashley Lyman, Pioneer in Pharmacy," *Pharm. Hist.* 14 (1972): 90–94, 111; Rufus A. Lyman, "Experimental Pharmacology: An Essential in the Pharmaceutical Curriculum," *Am. J. Pharm.* 82 (1910): 510–16; *Bulletin of the University of Nebraska: Annual Catalog of the School of Pharmacy,* 1910–11, pp. 13–14, 18.

73. Parascandola and Swann, "Pharmacology," pp. 97–99, 101–2.

74. Parascandola and Swann, "Pharmacology," pp. 104–9; A. Richard Bliss, "Pharmacodynamics in the Schools and Colleges of Pharmacy," *J. Am. Pharm. Assoc.* 9 (1920): 378–87; James Dille, "A Study of the Teaching of Pharmacology in Colleges of Pharmacy," *Am. J. Pharm. Educ.* 2 (1938): 8–31.

75. Herman G. Weiskotten et al., *Medical Education in the United States, 1934–1939* (Chicago: American Medical Association, 1940), p. 147.

76. Walter F. Riker, Jr. and Arthur H. Hayes, Jr., "A Viewpoint in Training Biomedical Scientists," in Aimo Pekkarinen, ed., *Contemporary Trends in the Training of Pharmacologists* (n.p.: International Union of Pharmacology, 1976), pp. 20–27, especially p. 21; Weiskotten et al., *Medical Education,* p. 148.

77. C. W. Edmunds, "The Teaching of Pharmacology," *J. Assoc. Am. Med. Coll.* 11 (1936): 83–93 (the quotation is from pp. 87–88).

78. Neil C. Moran, "Clinical Pharmacology—Old Wine in New Bottles," *Clin. Pharmacol. Ther.* 12 (1971): 417–26, especially p. 422.

79. William G. Van der Kloot, "The Education of Biomedical Scientists," in Judy Graves, ed., *The Future of Medical Education* (Durham, N.C.: Duke University Press, 1973), pp. 87–105 (the quotation is from p. 95).

80. A. C. Eycleshymer, "Report of Committee on Undergraduate and Graduate Degrees," *Proc. Assoc. Am. Med. Coll.* 29 (1919): 32–38, especially p. 36.

81. Weiskotten et al., *Medical Education,* p. 36.

82. Guy Stanton Ford, "An Experiment in Medical Graduate Work," *J. Assoc. Am. Med. Coll.* 5 (1930): 200–209, especially p. 208. J. Newell Stannard, "Zealous Companions in Research: The Graduate Studies Program," in *To Each His Farthest Star: University of Rochester Medical Center, 1925–1975* (Rochester, N.Y.: University of Rochester Medical Center, 1975), pp. 120–44.

83. *Cornell University Medical Bulletin: Announcement of the Medical College*, 1913, pp. 84–90; Henry Barbour to John Abel, 5 April 1917, Abel Papers, record group 1; *Bulletin of the University of Minnesota: Annual Register*, 1917–18, p. 135.

84. See the *Cornell University Medical Bulletin: Annual Announcement of the Medical College* and the *Bulletin of the University of Minnesota: Annual Register* for the period. The student who went on to earn a Ph.D at Chicago was John Quigley. See J. McKeen Cattell and Jacques Cattell, *American Men of Science*, 5th ed. (New York: Science Press, 1933), p. 905. The other two Minnesota students could not be found in sources such as *American Men of Science*, nor did they ever become members of the American Society for Pharmacology and Experimental Therapeutics. The entry on Minnesota in Vessell, *Survey of Pharmacology* pp. 445–52 states (p. 445) that the department granted its first Ph.D. in 1920, but I have not been able to confirm this claim in the medical school catalog.

85. On Tatum, see Parascandola and Keeney, *Sources*, pp. 52–53.

86. *University of Chicago, Circular of Information: Rush Medical College, Annual Announcement* for the period. On Van Dyke, see Parascandola and Keeney, *Sources*, pp. 54–55. On Nelson, see ibid., pp. 46–47.

87. Clark, *University of Wisconsin*, p. 103; Fisher and Carter, "Pharmacology at Tulane," p. 4.

88. William T. Salter, "Medicine as a Science: Pharmacology," *New England J. Med.* 244 (1951): 136–42, especially p. 137; *Graduate Training in Pharmacology*.

89. Riker and Hayes, "Viewpoint," p. 21, give the figures for 1952 as 45 percent Ph.D., 34 percent M.D., and 21 percent with both degrees; Julius H. Comroe, Jr. et al., "The Teaching of Physiology, Biochemistry, Pharmacology: Report of the First Teaching Institute, Association of American Medical Colleges, Atlantic City, October 19–23, 1953," *J. Med. Educ.* 29, no. 7, pt. 2 (1954) contains a table (p. 130) which gives the figures for 1953 as 51 percent Ph.D., 30 percent M.D., and 17 percent with both degrees (as well as 2 percent with neither degree).

90. A. R. McIntyre, "Flexner, Pharmacology and the Future," *J. Clin. Pharmacol.* 8 (1968): 278–80, especially p. 279.

91. Ibid., p. 279.

Chapter Five   Pharmacologists in Government and Industry

1. K. K. Chen, "Meetings," in K. K. Chen, ed., *The American Society for Pharmacology and Experimental Therapeutics, Incorporated: The First Sixty Years, 1908–1969* (Bethesda, Md.: American Society for Pharmacology and Experimental Therapeutics, 1969), pp. 1–119, especially pp. 6–7.

2. Victoria A. Harden, *Inventing the NIH: Federal Biomedical Research Policy, 1887–1937* (Baltimore: Johns Hopkins University Press, 1986),

pp. 3, 27–32; A. Hunter Dupree, *Science in the Federal Government: A History of Policies and Activities to 1940* (Cambridge: Harvard University Press, 1957), pp. 271–88.

3. Harden, *Inventing the NIH*, pp. 9–26.

4. Reid Hunt to Surgeon General Walter Wyman, 1 March 1904, General File (1897–1923), box 98, record group 90, National Archives, Washington, D.C. For biographical information on Hunt, see John Parascandola and Elizabeth Keeney, *Sources in the History of American Pharmacology* (Madison, Wis. American Institute of the History of Pharmacy, 1983), pp. 38–40; Eli Kennerly Marshall, "Reid Hunt, 1870–1948," *Biog. Mem. Natl. Acad. Sci.* 26 (1949): 25–49.

5. Reid Hunt, "Report of the Division of Pharmacology," in *Annual Report of the Surgeon-General of the Public Health and Marine-Hospital Service of the United States for the Fiscal Year 1905* (Washington, D.C.: Government Printing Office, 1906), pp. 226–27. After fiscal year 1911, the title of the annual report was changed to *Annual Report of the Surgeon General of the Public Health Service of the United States*.

6. Ramunas A. Kondratas, "Biologics Control Act of 1902," in *The Early Years of Federal Food and Drug Control* (Madison, Wis.: American Institute of the History of Pharmacy, 1982), pp. 8–27; Harden, *Inventing the NIH*, pp. 27–29.

7. On the movement for a food and drug act, see James Harvey Young, *Pure Food: Securing the Federal Food and Drugs Act of 1906* (Princeton: Princeton University Press, 1989).

8. On the *United States Pharmacopeia* and drug standards in America, see Glenn Sonnedecker, "Drug Standards become Official," in *Early Years of Federal Food and Drug Control*, pp. 28–39.

9. See the reports of the Division of Pharmacology in this period in *Annual Report of the Surgeon-General*.

10. Milton Rosenau, "General Report of the Director," in *Annual Report of the Surgeon-General*, 1906, p. 231.

11. *Annual Report of the Surgeon-General*, 1909, p. 71.

12. On the AMA's Council on Pharmacy and Chemistry, see Austin Smith, "The Council on Pharmacy and Chemistry and the Chemical Laboratory," In Morris Fishbein, ed., *A History of the American Medical Association, 1847–1947* (Philadelphia: W. B. Saunders, 1947), pp. 865–86.

13. See the reports of the division for this period in *Annual Report of the Surgeon-General*.

14. See the reports of the division in *Annual Report of the Surgeon-General*, 1906, p. 224; 1910, p. 55; 1911, p. 87; 1913, p. 55.

15. Ibid., 1905, p. 226.

16. Milton Rosenau to Surgeon General Walter Wyman, 3 March 1905, Public Health Service Records, RG 90, box 515, file S423, National Archives,

Washington, D.C. I am indebted to John Swann for calling my attention to this document.

17. See the reports of the division in this period in *Annual Report of the Surgeon General* and the bibliography of Hunt's publications in Marshall, "Reid Hunt," pp. 38–41.

18. Reid Hunt and R. de M. Taveau, "On the Physiological Action of Certain Cholin Derivatives and New Methods for Detecting Cholin," *Br. Med. J.*, (1906): 1788–91.

19. See the reports of the division in *Annual Report of the Surgeon General*, 1909, pp. 85–86; 1910, p. 53; 1900, p. 84.

20. *Annual Report of the Surgeon General*, 1910, pp. 53–56.

21. John Parascandola, "Carl Voegtlin and the 'Arsenic Receptor' in Chemotherapy," *J. Hist. Med.* 32 (1977): 151–71.

22. On the creation of NIH, see Harden, *Inventing the NIH*. On the activities of the Division of Pharmacology in the early NIH period, see the *Annual Report of the Surgeon General* for the 1930s.

23. On industrial toxicology and the work of the Public Health Service and the Bureau of Mines in this field, see Christopher Sellers, "The Public Health Service's Office of Industrial Hygiene and the Transformation of Industrial Medicine," *Bull. Hist. Med.* 65 (1991): 42–73; Christopher Sellers, "Manufacturing Disease: Experts and the Ailing American Worker" (Ph.D. diss., Yale University, 1992); Angela Nugent Young, "Interpreting the Dangerous Trades: Worker's Health in America and the Career of Alice Hamilton, 1910–1935" (Ph.D. diss., Brown University, 1981). On the tetraethyl lead conference, see "Proceedings of a Conference to Determine Whether or Not There is a Public Health Question in the Manufacture, Distribution or Use of Tetraethyl Lead Gasoline," *Public Health Bull.* (1925), vol. 158.

24. Lyman Kebler to John Abel, 17 March 1908, General Correspondence, box 210, class. no. 3242, record group 97, National Archives, Washington, D.C.

25. John Abel to Lyman Kebler, 18 March 1908, ibid.

26. Harvey Wiley, "1908 Report of Bureau of Chemistry," in *Federal Food, Drug and Cosmetic Law, Administrative Reports, 1907–1949* (Chicago: Commerce Clearing House, 1951), pp. 76–77; W. D. Bigelow to William Salant, 9 June 1908, General Correspondence, box 249, class. no. 15444, record group 97, National Archives, Washington, D.C.

27. On Salant, see Parascandola and Keeney, *Sources*, pp. 51–52.

28. See the annual reports of the bureau in this period in *Administrative Reports*.

29. For Wiley's efforts in these cases, see Oscar Anderson, *The Health of a Nation: Harvey W. Wiley and the Fight for Pure Food* (Chicago: University of Chicago Press, 1958), pp. 220–221, 235–37.

30. Harvey Wiley, "1911 Report of Bureau of Chemistry," in *Administrative Reports*, p. 223.

31. See James Whorton, *Before Silent Spring: Pesticides and Public Health in Pre-DDT America* (Princeton: Princeton University Press, 1974), pp. 144–45.

32. See W. Salant and J. B. Rieger, "The Elimination of Toxicity of Caffein in Nephrectomized Rabbits," *Proc. Soc. Exp. Biol. Med.* 9 (1912): 58–59; W. Salant and J. K. Phelps, "The Influence of Caffein on Protein Metabolism in Dogs, with Some Remarks on Demethylation in the Body," *J. Pharmacol. Exp. Ther.* 2 (1911): 401–2. Salant and his colleagues generally published only brief reports of their results in the "proceedings" of professional societies appearing in the journals associated with those bodies (as in the two cases cited here). Apparently they reserved fuller publication of their results for bulletins issued by the Bureau of Chemistry.

33. On Alsberg, see the biographical article by Mel Gorman in Wyndham Miles, ed., *American Chemists and Chemical Engineers* (Washington, D.C.: American Chemical Society, 1976), pp. 7–8.

34. Whorton, *Before Silent Spring*, pp. 142–60.

35. James Harvey Young, *The Medical Messiahs: A Social History of Health Quackery in Twentieth-Century America* (Princeton: Princeton University Press, 1967), p. 98.

36. Walter Campbell, "1935 Report of Food and Drug Administration," in *Federal Food, Drug and Cosmetic Law: Administrative Reports, 1907–1949* (Chicago: Commerce Clearing House, 1951), pp. 848–49 (pp. 24–25 of original report).

37. Oral History of the U.S. Food and Drug Administration: Pharmacology," transcription of a recording of a meeting to discuss the history of pharmacology in the Food and Drug Administration, Rockville, Md., 20 June 1980, History of Medicine Division, National Library of Medicine, Bethesda, Md. pp. 1–13 (the quotation is from p. 11). On Nelson, see Parascandola and Keeney, *Sources*, pp. 46–47. On the lead arsenate spray residue controversy, see Whorton, *Before Silent Spring*.

38. Walter Campbell, "1936 Report of Food and Drug Administration," in *Federal Food, Drug and Cosmetic Law*, p. 866 (p. 16 of original report).

39. On the 1938 act, see Charles O. Jackson, *Food and Drug Legislation in the New Deal* (Princeton: Princeton University Press, 1970). On Draize, see John Parascandola, "The Development of the Draize Test for Eye Toxicity," *Pharm. Hist.* 33 (1991): 111–17.

40. U. G. Houck, *The Bureau of Animal Industry of the United States Department of Agriculture: Its Establishment, Achievements and Current Activities* (Washington, D.C.: privately printed, 1924), pp. 79–82. On Crawford, see the biographical sketch in Parascandola and Keeney, *Sources*, p. 30.

41. Harden, *Inventing the NIH*, pp. 3, 27–32.

42. For general information on the Chemical Warfare Service, see Amos A. Fries and Clarence J. West, *Chemical Warfare* (New York: McGraw-Hill, 1921); Daniel P. Jones, "The Role of Chemists in Research on War Gases in the United States During World War I" (Ph.D. diss., University of Wisconsin–Madison, 1969). On the pharmacological and toxicological work, see Stephen A. Gross, "The Formation and Function of the Pharmacological and Toxicological Section, Research Division, Chemical Warfare Service, U.S. Army" (unpublished M.A. paper, Department of the History of Science, University of Wisconsin–Madison, 1982); H. C. Bradley, "Dr. Loevenhart's War Work," typescript, University of Wisconsin Medical School, Pharmacology and Toxicology Papers, University of Wisconsin–Madison Archives, Madison, ser. 12/14/5–1, box 1; A. C. Kolls, "History of Pharmacological and Toxicological Section, Research Division, Chemical Warfare Service, U.S. Army," ibid., ser. 12/14/9, box 4.

43. See John Parascandola, "Charles Holmes Herty and the Effort to Establish an Institute for Drug Research in Post World War I America," In John Parascandola and James C. Whorton, *Chemistry and Modern Society: Historical Essays in Honor of Aaron J. Ihde* (Washington, D.C.: American Chemical Society, 1983), pp. 85–103.

44. See John J. Beer, "Coal Tar Dye Manufacture and the Origins of the Modern Industrial Research Laboratory," *Isis* 49 (1958): 123–31; Georg Meyer-Thurow, "The Industrialization of Invention: A Case Study from the German Chemical Industry," *Isis* 73 (1982): 363–81.

45. On the early development of science and research in the American pharmaceutical industry, see Jonathan Liebenau, *Medical Science and Medical Industry: The Formation of the American Pharmaceutical Industry* (Baltimore: Johns Hopkins University Press, 1987), pp. 1–47; John P. Swann, *Academic Scientists and the Pharmaceutical Industry: Cooperative Research in Twentieth-Century America* (Baltimore: Johns Hopkins University Press, 1988), pp. 9–23; Malcolm Keith Weikel and Glenn Sonnedecker, "Emergence of Research as a Function of the American Pharmaceutical Industry" (unpublished manuscript, American Institute of the History of Pharmacy, Madison, Wis. 1963).

46. Liebenau, *Medical Science*, pp. 89–97; Sonnedecker, "Drug Standards," pp. 28–39.

47. This discussion of the early history of chemical and biological standardization efforts is based on Peter Stechl, "Biological Standardization of Drugs Before 1928" (Ph.D. diss., University of Wisconsin–Madison, 1969), pp. 1–45.

48. On Ehrlich and biological standardization of the diphtheria antitoxin, see ibid., pp. 46–58.

49. On these early research efforts at Parke-Davis, see ibid., pp. 60–65, 110–12; Weikel and Sonnedeker, "Emergence of Research," pp. 41–44.

50. Stechl, "Biological Standardization," pp. 60–65, 70–85, 110–12; Elijah M. Houghton, "Is Physiological Action Requisite as a Department of Pharmaceutical Research?" *Pharm. Era* 22 (1899): 399–400.

51. See letters from Parke-Davis to F. E. Stewart, 1884, Francis Edward Stewart Papers, box 7, Archives Division, State Historical Society of Wisconsin, Madison.

52. Liebenau, *Medical Science*, pp. 57–78; Stechl, "Biological Standardization," pp. 112–15; Joseph McFarland, "The Beginnings of Bacteriology in Philadelphia," *Bull. Hist. Med.* 5 (1937): 149–98, especially pp. 184–90; "Contract between H. K. Mulford Co., of Philadelphia, Pa., and Dr. Torald Sollmann, Cleveland, Ohio," 2-page typed document dated 21 March 1900, Torald Sollmann Papers, Historical Division, Cleveland Health Sciences Library, Cleveland.

53. Stechl, "Biological Standardization," pp. 114–19, 128; Jonathan Liebenau, "Medical Science and Medical Industry, 1890–1929: A Study of Pharmaceutical Manufacturing in Philadelphia" (Ph.D. diss., University of Pennsylvania, 1981), p. 406. For an example of Pittenger's work, see Paul S. Pittenger, *Biochemic Drug Assay Methods, with Special Reference to the Pharmacodynamic Standardization of Drugs* (Philadelphia: P. Blakiston's Son and Co., 1914).

54. Liebenau, "Pharmaceutical Manufacturing in Philadelphia," p. 422; "Who's Who in the H. K. Mulford Company: Francis E. Stewart, M.D.," *The Keystone* (published by H. K. Mulford Company, Philadelphia), vol. 2, no. 9, (November 1919), p. 1, copy in Stewart Papers, box 9.

55. Stechl, "Biological Standardization," pp. 110, 124–26; Horatio C. Wood, Jr., "Physiological Standardization: Its Value and Limitations," *Am. J. Pharm.* 82 (1910): 101–12; Horatio C. Wood, Jr., "The Purpose and Limitations of Bio-Assay," *J.A.M.A.* 59 (1912): 1433–34.

56. Kendall Birr, "The Roots of Industrial Research," in Harold Vagtborg, *Research and American Industrial Development: A Bicentennial Look at the Contribution of Applied R and D* (New York: Pergamon Press, 1976), pp. 24–50 (the quotation is from p. 40).

57. For a discussion of the growth of research in the American pharmaceutical industry in this period, see John Parascandola, "Industrial Research Comes of Age: The American Pharmaceutical Industry, 1920–1940," *Pharmacy in History* 27 (1985): 12–21. On the rise of cooperative research, see Swann, *Academic Scientists*.

58. Weikel and Sonnedecker, "Research," p. 48; *Lilly Research Laboratories, Dedication* (Indianapolis: Eli Lilly and Company, 1934), p. ix; "Physiological Testing Records," 1904–8, Eli Lilly and Company Archives, Indianapolis, Ind.; Gene E. McCormick to Glenn Sonnedecker, 10 June 1969, Kremers Reference Files, C38aI Lilly, F. B. Power Pharmaceutical Library, University of Wisconsin–Madison.

59. *The Lilly Scientific Bulletin*, ser. 1, no. 1, 16 April 1912, p. 2;

Charles R. Eckler Personnel Folder, Lilly Archives; Research Records, 1912–23, Lilly Archives. For examples of pharmacological publications, see C. R. Eckler, "Experiments with the Cat Method for Testing Digitalis and Its Allies," *Am. J. Pharm.* 83 (1911): 478–91; Charles R. Eckler, "Apparatus for Studying the Effect of Drugs on the Isolated Guinea Pig Uterus," *J. Lab. Clin. Med.* 2 (1917): 819–24.

60. See Arthur L. Walters and E. W. Koch, "Pharmacological Studies of the Ipecac Alkaloids and Some Synthetic Derivatives of Cephaeline. I. Studies on Toxicity," *J. Pharmacol. Exp. Ther.* 10 (1917): 73–81. For information on the authors, see Arthur L. Walters Personnel Folder, Lilly Archives; the biographical sketch on Koch in J. McKeen Cattell and Jacques Cattell, *American Men of Science: A Biographical Directory,* 5th ed. (New York: Science Press, 1933), p. 628.

61. E. J. Kahn, Jr., *All in a Century: The First 100 Years of Eli Lilly and Company* (n.p., [1976]), pp. 92–101; Swann, *Academic Scientists,* pp. 38–40, 118–69. For biographical information on Clowes, see M. E. Krahl, "George Henry Alexander Clowes, 1877–1958," *Cancer Res.* 19 (1959): 334–36.

62. Letter from G. H. A. Clowes to C. W. McCoy, 9 October 1919, Lilly Archives. Part of the letter is reproduced in Kahn, *All in a Century,* pp. 93–94.

63. Typescript of interview of K. K. Chen and Charles L. Rose by Gene E. McCormick, 6 and 16 February 1968, Lilly Archives, pp. 2–9; "Dr. Chen Joins Lilly Staff," *Tile and Till* 16 (January 1930): 14, copy in Lilly Archives; K. K. Chen, "Remington Address: In Pursuit of Science," *J. Am. Pharm. Assoc.* NS6 (1966): 27–28; biographical form filled out by K. K. Chen, Kremers Reference Files, A2 section (Chen), F. B. Power Pharmaceutical Library, University of Wisconsin–Madison.

64. John Parascandola, "Industrial Research Comes of Age: The American Pharmaceutical Industry, 1920–1940," *Pharm. Hist* 27 (1985): 12–21, especially pp. 15–16; Swann, *Academic Scientists,* p. 68; memorandum from R. T. Major to Mr. Robertson, 8 April 1932, Merck and Company Archives, Rahway, N.J.

65. Swann, *Academic Scientists,* pp. 66–70; A. N. Richards to George W. Perkins, 23 September 1930, Alfred N. Richards Papers, box 32, University of Pennsylvania Archives, Philadelphia.

66. A. N. Richards to Hallowell Davis, 15 December 1931; A. N. Richards to E. P. Pick, 18 December 1931; A. N. Richards to Lafayette Mendel, 8 January 1932; A. N. Richards to Hans Molitor, 6 May 1932; Richards Papers, box 30. Swann, *Academic Scientists,* pp. 70–74.

67. Swann, *Academic Scientists,* pp. 43–45; F. J. Kessler, typescript entitled "Merck Sharpe & Dohme Research Laboratories, Historical Sketch," 20 January 1982, Merck and Company Archives.

68. Hans Molitor to A. N. Richards, 2 December 1938; Merck Institute

of Therapeutic Research, Third Annual Report to the Board of Trustees, by Hans Molitor, M.D., Director, 15 January 1936; Sixth Annual Report (1938), Merck Institute of Therapeutic Research; Richards Papers, box 30.

69. Merck Institute, Third Annual Report.

70. A. N. Richards, E. K. Marshall, Jr., 26 September 1932; A. N. Richards, to H. S. Gasser, 6 June 1934; Chauncey Leake to Hans Molitor, 27 April 1936; Richards Papers, box 30.

71. Chauncey Leake to Hans Molitor, 27 April 1936, Richards Papers, box 30.

72. Sinclair Lewis, *Arrowsmith* (New York: Harcourt Brace, 1925), p. 137.

73. Ellsworth Cook, "Revisions of the Constitution and Bylaws," in Chen, ed., *American Society*, pp. 175–77, 184.

74. Undated draft of a letter from Reid Hunt to a committee of the Council of the American Society for Pharmacology and Experimental Therapeutics appointed to draw up a constitution and bylaws, copy attached to a letter from Hunt to John Abel, 2 January 1909, Abel Papers, record group 1. The Abel Papers also contain a revised draft of this committee letter (also undated), and it includes the same statement.

75. Ibid. The initial draft named only Hunt, Crawford, and Abel, but the revised draft added Loevenhart.

76. See the correspondence on ASPET origins in the C. W. Edmunds Files, American Society for Pharmacology and Experimental Therapeutics Archives, Bethesda, Md.; the minutes of the organizational (1908) and first annual (1909) meeting of ASPET, Minutes and Records, vol. 1 (1908–1916), ibid.; the extensive correspondence on the founding of the society in the Abel Papers, record group 1.

77. The Association of Official Agricultural Chemists did not admit industrial chemists, but there was no explicit ban in their constitution against such individuals. The association only accepted as active members chemists associated with one of three types of institutions: the United States Department of Agriculture; any national, state, or provincial experiment station or college engaged in agricultural chemistry research; and any national, state, or provincial body charged with the official control of fertilizers, feeds, and other agricultural products. Industrial chemists were not singled out for exclusion. Chemists who worked for municipal laboratories or private research foundations, for example, were also ineligible to become active members. See Association of Official Agricultural Chemists, *Golden Anniversary of the Association of Official Agricultural Chemists, 1884–1934* (Washington, D.C.: [1934]), p. 19.

78. Charles Browne and Mary Weeks, *A History of the American Chemical Society: Seventy-five Eventful Years* (Washington, D.C.: American Chemical Society, 1952); Herman Skolnick and Kenneth Reese, eds., *A Century*

of Chemistry: The Role of Chemists and the American Chemical Society (Washington, D.C.: American Chemical Society, 1976).

79. American Physiological Society, *History of the American Physiological Society, Semicentennial, 1887–1937* (Baltimore: 1938); John Brobeck, Orr Reynolds, and Toby Appel, *History of the American Physiological Society: The First Century, 1887–1937* (Bethesda, Md.: American Physiological Society, 1987); Russell H. Chittenden, *The First Twenty-five Years of the American Society for Biological Chemists* (New Haven: American Society of Biological Chemists, 1945).

80. On patent medicine quackery in this period, see James Harvey Young, *The Toadstool Millionaires: A Social History of Patent Medicines in America before Federal Regulation* (Princeton: Princeton University Press, 1961).

81. John Abel to Robert Hatcher, 31 January 1910, Abel Papers, record group 1.

82. John Abel to L. R. Hudson, 7 December 1915, Abel Papers, record group 1.

83. For a discussion of this point, see Swann, *Academic Scientists*, pp. 30–32.

84. For information on membership, see the society histories cited in notes 1, 78, and 79 to this chapter.

85. Robert Hatcher to Arthur Loevenhart, 26 December 1919, Arthur Loevenhart Papers, box 3, University of Wisconsin Archives, Madison.

86. Torald Sollmann to John Abel, 9 February 1927, Abel Papers, record group 1. Abel himself commented that "for reasons evident to all medical men, it is the intention of the founders to impose unusual restrictions upon its members in respect to their connection with drug firms and other industrial concerns, a step that has my unqualified approval." John Abel to Edmund James, 5 January 1909, ibid.

87. Samuel Meltzer to John Abel, 31 October 1910, Abel Papers, record group 1.

88. Reid Hunt to John Abel, 28 February 1927, Abel Papers, record group 1.

89. Minutes of the fifth (1913) annual meeting of ASPET, Minutes and Records, vol. 1 (1908–1916), ASPET Archives.

90. Francis Stewart to Edward Kremers, 21 February 1918, Kremers Reference Files, A2 section (Stewart), F. B. Power Pharmaceutical Library, University of Wisconsin–Madison; John Abel to Irvine Page, 3 November 1926, Abel Papers, record group 1.

91. John Abel, "The Methods of Pharmacology, with Experimental Illustration," *Pharm. Era* 7 (1892): 105.

92. John Abel to William deB. MacNider, 5 April 1935, Abel Papers, record group 1.

93. John Abel to Edmund James, 5 January 1909 and John Abel to A. P. Matthews, 4 January 1909, Abel Papers, record group 1.

94. John Abel to Arthur Cushny, 25 January 1916, Abel Papers, record group 1.

95. Arthur Loevenhart to Abel, 28 January 1918, 14 March 1919, 9 January 1920 and C. W. Edmunds to Abel, 6 March 1919, 9 January 1920, 5 January 1921, Abel Papers, record group 1; minutes of eleventh (1919) and twelfth (1920) annual meetings of ASPET, Minutes and Records, vol. 2 (1917–1927), ASPET Archives.

96. C. W. Edmunds to John Abel, 5 January 1921 and John Abel to C. W. Edmunds, 10 January 1921, Abel Papers, record group 1.

97. I have discussed the development of research in the American pharmaceutical industry during this period in other publications. See John Parascandola, "Industrial Research Comes of Age: The American Pharmaceutical Industry, 1920–1940," *Pharmacy in History* 27 (1985): 12–21. See also Swann, *Academic Scientists*, pp. 9–56.

98. John Abel to Reid Hunt, 25 January 1927, Abel Papers, record group 1.

99. John Abel to Torald Sollmann, 2 February 1927, Abel Papers, record group 1.

100. For a discussion of the growing interaction between academic scientists and the pharmaceutical industry in this period, see Swann, *Academic Scientists*.

101. Ibid., pp. 93–117. See also John Swann, "Arthur Tatum, Parke-Davis, and the Discovery of Mapharsen as an Antisyphilitic Agent," *J. Hist. Med.* 40 (1985): 167–87.

102. Swann, *Academic Scientists*, pp. 65–86.

103. Robert Hatcher to John Abel, 28 January 1910; A. N. Richards to John Abel, 30 August 1930; William deB. MacNider to John Abel, 29 May 1931; Abel Papers, record group 1.

104. Swann, *Academic Scientists*, p. 75.

105. See "Proposed Amendment to the Constitution of the American Society for Pharmacology and Experimental Therapeutics," undated printed document, minutes of twelfth (1920) annual meeting of ASPET, Minutes and Records, vol. 2 (1917–27), ASPET Archives. A copy of this proposed amendment from the 1920 meeting is also attached to a letter from Arthur Hirschfelder to John Abel, 20 January 1927, Abel Papers, record group 1.

106. Arthur Loevenhart to John Abel, 14 March 1919, Abel Papers, record group 1.

107. See Robert Hatcher to John Abel, 4 February 1927, Abel Papers, record group 1.

108. Ibid.

109. Torald Sollmann to John Abel, 9 February 1927; John Abel to Arthur

Loevenhart, 16 February 1927; John Abel to David Macht, 1 March 1927; David Macht to John Abel, 2 March 1927; John Abel to Chauncey Leake, 22 March 1932; Abel Papers, record group 1.

110. Minutes of the twentieth (1929) annual meeting of ASPET, Minutes and Records, vol. 3 (1928–34), ASPET Archives.

111. David Macht to Simon Flexner, 25 October 1928, Simon Flexner Papers, American Philosophical Society, Philadelphia.

112. David Macht to Simon Flexner, 12 January 1927, Flexner Papers.

113. Henry Dale to A. N. Richards, 6 April 1933, Richards Papers, box 32. I am grateful to John Swann for calling my attention to this letter.

114. A. N. Richards to ASPET Council, 4 April 1935, Richards Papers, box 10.

115. E. M. K. Geiling to A. N. Richards, 26 April 1936, Richards Papers, box 10; minutes of the twenty-sixth (1935) annual meeting of the ASPET Council, Minutes and Records, vol. 4 (1935–37), ASPET Archives.

116. E. M. K. Geiling to ASPET members, 16 January 1937, Minutes and Records, vol. 4 (1935–1937), ASPET Archives.

117. Minutes of the twenty-seventh (1936) annual meeting of ASPET, Minutes and Records, vol. 4 (1935–37), ASPET Archives.

118. Minutes of the twenty-eighth (1937) annual meeting of ASPET, Minutes and Records, vol. 4 (1935–37), ASPET Archives.

119. Harry Van Dyke to Charles Gruber, 14 July 1938 and Harry Van Dyke to G. Philip Grabfield, 21 November 1938, appended to the minutes of the thirtieth (1939) annual meeting of ASPET Council, Minutes and Records, vol. 5 (1938–39), ASPET Archives.

120. Arthur Tatum to G. Grabfield, 22 July 1938, Arthur Tatum Papers, box 2, University of Wisconsin Archives, Madison.

121. Minutes of the thirtieth (1939) annual meeting of ASPET Council, Minutes and Records, vol. 5 (1938–39), ASPET Archives.

122. Petition to G. Grabfield, 6 November 1940, Minutes and Records, vol. 6 (1940–41), ASPET Archives.

123. Minutes of the thirty-second (1941) annual meeting of ASPET, Minutes and Records, vol. 6 (1940–41), ASPET Archives.

124. Swann, *Academic Scientists*, pp. 170–81, (the quotation is from p. 181).

Chapter Six   The Professionalization of a Discipline

1. Robert E. Kohler, *From Medical Chemistry to Biochemistry: The Making of a Biomedical Discipline* (Cambridge: Cambridge University Press, 1982), p. 196.

2. John T. Edsall, "The Journal of Biological Chemistry After Seventy-five Years," *J. Biol. Chem.* 255 (1980): 8939–51 (the quotation is from p. 8940).

The Abel Papers contain a significant amount of material on the founding and early history of the journal, particularly in Abel's correspondence with C. A. Herter and A. N. Richards in the period 1903 to 1909 (record group 1). Some of these materials are cited in succeeding notes.

3. Christian Herter to John Abel, 24 May 1903, Abel Papers, record group 1.

4. Edsall, "Journal," pp. 8939–40.

5. Kohler, *Medical Chemistry*, pp. 199–202; Russell H. Chittenden, *The First Twenty-five Years of the American Society of Biological Chemists* (New Haven: American Society of Biological Chemists, 1945), pp. 1–8.

6. Typescript of an address for the meeting of the Federation of American Societies for Experimental Biology, Montreal, 10 April 1931, Abel Papers, record group 6. A handwritten note by Abel indicates that he did not actually read this text at the meeting, but spoke "off hand," and that he deleted the section about the pregnancy of the Physiological Society and his serving as a midwife to the birth of new groups.

7. Letter from John Abel to various biochemists, 13 December 1906, Abel Papers, record group 1.

8. Torald Sollmann to John Abel, 17 December 1906, Abel Papers, record group 1.

9. Robert Hatcher to John Abel, 18 December 1906 and George Wallace to John Abel, 18 December 1906, Abel Papers, record group 1.

10. William Gies to John Abel, 23 December 1906, Abel Papers, record group 1.

11. Chittenden, *First Twenty-five Years*, pp. 40–42.

12. John Abel to Torald Sollmann, 9 January 1907, William de Berniere MacNider Papers, Southern Historical Collections, North Carolina Library, Chapel Hill, box 1, folder 1.

13. George Wallace to John Abel, 4 December 1907, Abel Papers, record group 1; John Abel to Torald Sollmann, 16 January 1908, MacNider Papers, box 1, folder 1.

14. John Abel to Torald Sollmann, 16 January 1908, MacNider Papers, box 1, folder 1. George H. Simmons was the editor of the *Journal of the American Medical Association* at the time.

15. Untitled, undated typescript invitation to organizational meeting, Abel Papers, record group 1. Although this document is undated, it would appear from the many responses dated around mid-December 1908 (Abel Papers, record group 1) that it was sent in the first half of that month.

16. "Minutes of a Meeting Called to Organize the American Society for Pharmacology and Experimental Therapeutics," typescript, Minutes and Records, vol. 1, American Society for Pharmacology and Experimental Therapeutics Archives, Bethesda, Md. (copy also in Abel Papers, record group 1); copy of "Articles of Agreement" of the American Society of Biological Chemists

with handwritten changes by John Abel modifying it for use by the American Society for Pharmacology and Experimental Therapeutics, Abel Papers, record group 1; K. K. Chen, ed., *The American Society for Pharmacology and Experimental Therapeutics, Incorporated: The First Sixty Years 1908–1969* (Bethesda, Md.: The American Society for Pharmacology and Experimental Therapeutics, 1969), pp. 5–11. The founders, and their institutional affiliations at the time, were: John Abel (Johns Hopkins University), Carl Alsberg (Bureau of Plant Industry, United States Department of Agriculture [USDA]), John Auer (Rockefeller Institute), Albert Crawford, (Bureau of Animal Industry, USDA), Charles Edmunds (University of Michigan), J. A. English Eyster (University of Virginia), W. Worth Hale (Hygienic Laboratory, United States Public Health Service [USPHS]), Robert Hatcher (Cornell University), Velyien Henderson (University of Toronto), Reid Hunt (Hygienic Laboratory, USPHS), Arthur Loevenhart (University of Wisconsin), Samuel Mathews (University of Chicago), Samuel Meltzer (Rockefeller Institute), William Salant (Bureau of Chemistry, USDA), Torald Sollmann (Western Reserve University), Maurice Tyrode (Harvard University), Carl Voegtlin (Johns Hopkins University), and Horatio C. Wood, Jr. (University of Pennsylvania). For more information on the founders, see Chen, *American Society*.

17. "The American Pharmacologic Society and the Working Bulletin System for the Collective Investigation of the Newer Materia Medica," 6-page typescript, [1906]; F. E. Stewart, *Prospectus of the American Pharmacologic Society and the Working Bulletin System for the Co-Operative Investigation of New Materia Medica and Food-Products* (New York: American Pharmacologic Society, 1906), advance proofs; Francis Edward Stewart Papers, box 12, Archives Division, State Historical Society of Wisconsin, Madison.

18. Torald Sollmann, "The Early Days of the Pharmacological Society" (paper presented at the meeting of the American Society for Pharmacology and Experimental Therapeutics, Detroit, 21 April 1949), in James W. Fisher, ed., *Readings on the History of Pharmacology* (New Orleans: Tulane University Department of Pharmacology, 1971), pp. 56–58. On Ehrlich and experimental therapeutics, see John Parascandola, "The Theoretical Basis of Paul Ehrlich's Chemotherapy," *J. Hist. Med.* 36 (1981): 19–43.

19. Torald Sollmann to John Abel, 6 November 1908; Abel Papers, record group 1; Samuel Meltzer to Charles Edmunds, 1 February 1909, Correspondence, ASPET Origins, C. W. Edmunds Files, ASPET Archives.

20. Albert Mathews to John Abel, 22 November 1908, Abel Papers, record group 1. In this letter, Mathews discussed his own department, and agreed with Abel that physiology, biochemistry, and pharmacology should not be combined as they were at Chicago, but should be independent departments. The only difficulty he saw in this approach at Chicago was in "keeping the pharmacology out of the clutches of the clinical men."

21. Albert Mathews to John Abel, 9 December 1908, Abel Papers, record group 1.

22. Carl Alsberg to Charles Edmunds, 1 April 1909, Correspondence, ASPET Origins, C. W. Edmunds Files, ASPET Archives.

23. Charles Edmunds to John Abel, 18 January 1909 and Reid Hunt to John Abel, 25 January 1909, Abel Papers, record group 1; Samuel Meltzer to Charles Edmunds, 1 February 1909 and Reid Hunt to Charles Edmunds, 15 March 1909, Correspondence, ASPET Origins, C. W. Edmunds Files, ASPET Archives.

24. Gerald Geison, "Divided We Stand: Physiologists and Clinicians in the American Context," in Morris Vogel and Charles Rosenberg, eds., *The Therapeutic Revolution: Essays in the Social History of American Medicine* (Philadelphia: University of Pennsylvania Press, 1979), pp. 67–90 (the quotation is from p. 67); Russell Maulitz, " 'Physician Versus Bacteriologist:' The Ideology of Science in Clinical Medicine," ibid., pp. 91–107. See also John Parascandola, "The Search for the Active Oxytocic Principle of Ergot: Laboratory Science and Clinical Medicine in Conflict," in Erika Hickel and Gerald Schröder, eds., *Neue Beiträge zur Arzneimittelgeschichte: Festschrift für Wolfgang Schneider zum 70. Geburtstag* (Stuttgart: Wissenschaftliche Verlagsgesellschaft, 1982), *Veröff. Int. Ges. Gesch. Pharm.*, n.s. 51: 205–27.

25. Torald Sollmann to Charles Edmunds, 15 March 1909; Samuel Meltzer to Charles Edmunds, 15 March 1909; Reid Hunt to Charles Edmunds, 31 January 1909; Correspondence, ASPET Origins, C. W. Edmunds Files, ASPET Archives. Torald Sollmann to John Abel, 25 January 1909, Abel papers, record group 1.

26. Chen, *American Society*, pp. 11, 15.

27. Typewritten draft of constitution, Correspondence, ASPET Origins, C. W. Edmunds Files, ASPET Archives; Ellsworth Cook, "Revision of the Constitutions and Bylaws," in Chen, *American Society*, pp. 175–196.

28. Chen, *American Society*, pp. 11–17; minutes of the first annual meeting, 1909, Minutes and Records, vol. 1 (1908–16), ASPET Archives.

29. On the growth in membership of the society, see Allan D. Bass, "Growth," in Chen, *American Society*, pp. 155–72, especially pp. 158–59.

30. John Herter to C. A. Abel, 24 September, 12 November 1907, Abel Papers, record group 1.

31. Untitled, undated invitation to organizational meeting; Certificate of Incorporation of the Journal of Pharmacology and Experimental Therapeutics Society, Incorporated; Constitution and Bylaws of the Journal of Pharmacology and Experimental Therapeutics Society, Incorporated, Abel Papers, record group 1.

32. *Three Quarters of a Century plus Ten, 1890–1975* (Baltimore: Waverly Press, 1975), pp. 12–13; *The Kalends of the Williams and Wilkins Company*, 4, no. 2 (1925): 1; John T. Edsall, "The Journal of Biological Chemistry

after Seventy-five Years," *J. Biol. Chem.* 255 (1980): 8939–51, especially p. 8940.

33. Announcement of the *Journal of Pharmacology and Experimental Therapeutics*, undated, Abel Papers, record group 1.

34. Ibid.

35. *J. Pharmacol. Exp. Ther.* 1 (1909–10).

36. These data were obtained from a count of the articles in the *Journal of Pharmacology and Experimental Therapeutics* for the period. In the cases of papers submitted by authors from more than one department or institution, the credit was split (e.g., one-half paper was credited to each department in the case of a paper coauthored by two scientists from different departments). The data were compiled by John Swann while he was working under my direction as a research assistant at the University of Wisconsin–Madison, with support from NIH grant LM 03300 from the National Library of Medicine.

37. W. F. Bynum, *An Early History of the British Pharmacological Society* (London: British Pharmacological Society, 1981).

38. C. A. Herter to John Abel, 15 December 1908, Abel Papers, record group 1.

39. Letters to John Abel dated 18 December 1911 from Robert Hatcher, Reid Hunt, A. S. Loevenhart, and S. J. Meltzer and dated 19 December 1911 from C. W. Edmunds. Torald Sollmann, and George Wallace, Abel Papers, record group 1; Bynum, *British Pharmacological Society*, p. 4; Maurice H. Seevers, "Publications," in Chen, ed., *American Society*, pp. 123–36, especially pp. 127–28.

40. John Abel to Henry Barbour, 30 June 1922, to Robert Hatcher, 21 and 26 July 1922, to Carl Alsberg, 7 October 1922, to John Murlin, 9 June 1931; Walter Dixon to John Abel, 3 July 1926; Abel Papers, record group 1.

41. Robert Hatcher to John Abel, 24 July 1922; John Abel to Robert Hatcher, 26 July 1922, 17 June 1930; Abel to A. D. Hirschfelder, 11 February 1930; Abel to Murlin, 9 June 1931; Abel to Alsberg, 7 October 1922; Abel Papers, record group 1.

42. John Abel to David Macht, 9 January 1928, to Robert Hatcher, 17 June 1930, to Kenneth Melville, 23 October 1930, Abel Papers, record group 1.

43. John Abel to Attilo Rizzolo, 20 July 1929, Abel Papers, record group 1.

44. John Abel to H. V. Atkinson, 24 March 1928, Abel Papers, record group 1.

45. G. E. Farrar, Jr. and A. M. Duff, Jr., "Ergotamine Tartrate: Its Direct Hyperglycemic Action and Its Influence on the Hyperglycemia Produced by Epinephrine in Normal Unanesthetized Dogs," *J. Pharmacol. Exp. Ther.* 34 (1928): 197–202 (the quotation is from p. 198); H. V. Atkinson, "The

Effect of External and Internal Application of Heat and Cold on the Muscular Activity of the Stomach in Unanesthetized Dogs," ibid., 33 (1928): 321–27.

46. John Abel to Sanford Rosenthal, 12 November 1929 and Sanford Rosenthal to John Abel, 27 November 1929, Abel Papers, record group 1; Sanford M. Rosenthal, "Some Effects of Alcohol upon the Normal and Damaged Liver," *J. Pharmacol. Exp. Ther.* 38 (1930): 291–301 (the table in question is on p. 295).

47. Susan Lederer, "Political Animals: Biomedical Research Journalism and Animal Experimentation in Twentieth-Century America," *Isis* 83 (1992): 61–79.

48. Copy of letter from John Abel to A. D. White, 3 August 1914; Abel to Edward Passano, 3 March 1915, to George Simmons, 14 and 24 January 1916; George Simmons to John Abel, 7 and 18 January, 1916; Abel Papers, record group 1.

49. John Abel to D. O. Wilkinson, 25 January 1929, Abel Papers, record group 1.

50. John Abel to Reid Hunt, 19 April 1932, to Robert M. Lester, 7 June 1935, 19 September 1936, Abel papers, record group 1.

51. Carl Voegtlin, "John Jacob Abel, 1857–1938," *J. Pharmacol. Exp. Ther.* 67 (1939): 373–406, especially p. 399; William deBerniere MacNider, "Biographical Memoir of John Jacob Abel, 1857–1938," *Biog. Mem. Natl. Acad. Sci.* 24 (1947): 231–57, especially pp. 247–48; John J. Abel, "On Poisons and Disease and Some Experiments with the Toxin of the Bacillus Tetani," *Science* 79 (1934): 63–70, 121–29.

52. John Abel to S. J. Weinberg, 6 February 1936; John Abel to Mrs. Julius Y. Talmadge, 27 February 1937; John Abel to Reinhard Beutner, 19 May 1937; Abel Papers, record group 1.

53. John Abel to Mary Abel, 30 September [1931], Abel Papers, record group 1.

54. Voegtlin, "John Jacob Abel," p. 400; MacNider, "John Jacob Abel," pp. 231, 246; Warfield M. Firor, "John Jacob Abel, Retirement, 1932–1938," *Bull. Johns Hopkins Hosp.* 101 (1957): 327–28.

55. On Marshall, see Thomas H. Maren, "Eli Kennerly Marshall, Jr., 1889–1966," *Pharmacologist* 8 (1966): 90–94.

56. Chen, "Meetings," pp. 36–37; Seevers, "Publications"; Edward Passano to John Abel, 12 January 1933 and John Abel to Charles Edmunds, 2 June 1932, Abel Papers, record group 1; minutes of the twenty-fourth annual meeting of the American Society for Pharmacology and Experimental Therapeutics, 9 to 12 April 1933, Minutes and Records, vol. 3, ASPET Archives.

57. Maurice H. Seevers, "Projection to the Future," in Chen, ed., *American Society*, pp. 207–20, especially pp. 209–10; letter from Carl Cori to Alan Gregg, 28 October 1939 and letter from Torald Sollmann to Alan Gregg, 30 October 1939, Rockefeller Foundation Archives, RG2 200, American Medical Schools—Pharmacology, 1939, Rockefeller Archive Center, North Tar-

rytown, N. Y.; Herman G. Weiskotten et al., *Medical Education in the United States, 1934–1939* (Chicago: American Medical Association, 1940), pp. 147–49.

58. Alan Gregg, "Addenda to the Agenda for the Decade 1940–1950," *J. Amer. Med. Assoc.* 114 (1940): 1139–41 (the quotation is from p. 1140). In 1939 Gregg solicited letters from a number of American pharmacologists, asking for information on their programs and any comments that they might have that would "tend to approve the general thesis that pharmacology needs more attention than it is getting" (17 October 1939). A copy of Gregg's letter and the responses received may be found in the Rockefeller Foundation Archives, RG2 200, American Medical Schools—Pharmacology, 1939.

59. James Harvey Young, *The Medical Messiahs: A Social History of Health Quackery in Twentieth-Century America* (Princeton: Princeton University Press, 1967), p. 260.

60. *Graduate Training in Pharmacology Programs in the United States and Canada* (Bethesda, Md: American Society for Pharmacology and Experimental Therapeutics, 1988).

61. "New Members," *Pharmacologist*, 33 (1991): 101–3.

62. Gary O. Rankin, "Report on the Second Survey of the Subcommittee on Pharmacology Utilization and Training (SPUT) of ASPET," *Pharmacologist* 32 (1990): 230–35.

63. On clinical pharmacology, see Harry Gold, "Clinical Pharmacology—Historical Note," *J. Clin. Pharmacol. New Drugs* 7 (1967): 309–11; "Ninety Years of Therapeutics: A History of the American Society for Clinical Pharmacology and Therapeutics," *Clin. Pharmacol. Ther.* suppl., 47 (1990): 251–304. On clinical pharmacology in the medical curriculum, see David L. Cowen, "Materia Medica and Pharmacology," in Ronald L. Numbers, ed., *The Education of American Physicians: Historical Essays* (Berkeley: University of California Press, 1980), pp. 95–121, especially pp. 118–20.

64. Alexander M. M. Shepherd, "American Board of Clinical Pharmacology, Inc.: A Personal Commentary," *Pharmacologist* 32 (1990): 247–48.

65. On receptor theory, see John Parascandola, "The Development of Receptor Theory," In M. J. Parnhams and J. Bruinvels, eds., *Discoveries in Pharmacology* (Amsterdam: Elsevier, 1985), 3: 129–56.

66. Cowen, "Materia Medica and Pharmacology," p. 112. For an example of a biochemical breakthrough, the antimetabolite concept, and the enthusiasm that it generated, see D. W. Wooley, "The Revolution in Pharmacology," *Perspect. Biol. Med.* 1 (1958): 174–97.

67. On the development of molecular biology, see Horace F. Judson, *The Eighth Day of Creation: Makers of the Revolution in Biology* (New York: Simon and Schuster, 1979); Robert Olby, *The Path to the Double Helix* (Seattle: University of Washington Press, 1974).

68. Avram Goldstein, "The Three-Dimensional Structure of Pharmacology," *Pharmacologist* 23 (1981): 280–85 (the quotation is on p. 283).

69. William W. Fleming, "John V. Croker Memorial Lecture: The Im-

pact of Cell and Molecular Biology on Pharmacology," *Pharmacologist* 30 (1988): 146–48 (the quotation is on p. 147).

70. Goldstein, "Three-Dimensional Structure," pp. 283–84. For another recent example of a pharmacologist praising the breadth of the field, "ranging from molecular biology to clinical applications," see James A. Bain, "The 1988 Torald Sollmann Award Oration," *Pharmacologist* 31 (1989): 25–33 (the quotation is from p. 33).

71. John Parascandola, "Historical Perspectives on In Vitro Toxicology," *Alt. Meth. Toxicol.* 8 (1991): 87–96.

72. "Apathy of Bioscientists on Issues Surrounding Animals," *Pharmacologist* 24 (1982): 26.

73. Fleming, "Croker Memorial Lecture," p. 147.

74. Goldstein, "Three-Dimensional Structure," p. 284.

75. John Abel to Abraham Flexner, 3 July 1924, Abel Papers, record group 1.

BIBLIOGRAPHICAL ESSAY

The purpose of this bibliographical essay is not to list all of the sources consulted in this study (which are more exhaustively covered in the chapter notes), but to guide the reader to the most useful sources of information on the major subject areas discussed in the book. Readers are also advised to consult an earlier bibliographical publication coauthored by Elizabeth Keeney and myself, *Sources in the History of American Pharmacology* (Madison: American Institute of the History of Pharmacy, 1983), particularly for the biographical sketches of twenty-six selected American pharmacologists.

The Development of Pharmacology in Europe

Although this book is concerned with American pharmacology, the European background is essential to the story, and the reader is referred here to useful secondary literature on this subject. There is no scholarly, comprehensive history of pharmacology. Chauncey Leake's *An Historical Account of Pharmacology to the Twentieth Century* (Springfield, Ill.: Charles C Thomas, 1975) is not really a history of the science of pharmacology, even for the period purportedly covered (to 1900). About two-thirds of the book is devoted to knowledge about drugs in the period before pharmacology emerged as a discipline (or to what Leake calls "protopharmacology"), and the work is diffuse, anecdotal, and poorly documented. Only brief attention is given to such key figures in the emergence of the discipline as Magendie, Buchheim, and Schmiedeberg.

Readings in Pharmacology, B. Holmstedt and G. Liljestrand, eds. (Oxford: Pergamon Press, 1963), is basically a source book that can serve to a limited extent as an introduction to the history of the field. The biographical sketches of pharmacologists and the excerpts from their works (translated into English where necessary) are too brief, however, to do more than provide an entry into the subject. Louis Schuster, ed., *Readings in Pharmacology* (Boston: Little, Brown and Co., 1962), is also a source book. It provides many fewer readings than the Holmstedt and Liljestrand volume, but the papers are in most cases reproduced in their entirety (translated into English where necessary).

Melvin Earles's doctoral dissertation, "Studies in the Development of Experimental Pharmacology in the Eighteenth and Early Nineteenth Centuries" (University College, London, 1961), is still a useful source of information on early pharmacology. See also the following papers by Earles: "Experiments with Drugs and Poisons in the Seventeenth and Eighteenth Centuries," *Ann. Sci.* 19 (1963): 241–54; "Early Theories of the Mode of Action of Drugs and Poisons,"*Ann. Sci.* 17 (1961): 93–110; "The Experimental Investigations of Viper Venom by Felice Fontana (1730–1805)," *Ann. Sci.* 16 (1960): 255–68. On Fontana, see also P. K. Knoefel, "Felice Fontana on Poisons," *Clio Med.* 15 (1980): 35–65. On the history of the term *pharmacology*, see Gert Preiser, "Zum Geschichte und Bildung der Termini Pharmakologie und Toxikologie," *Medizinhist. J.* 2 (1967): 124–34.

On the beginnings of experimental pharmacology in France, see John Lesch, *Science and Medicine in France: The Emergence of Experimental Physiology, 1790–1855* (Cambridge: Harvard University Press, 1984). J. M. D. Olmsted's biography, *François Magendie* (New York: Schumann's, 1944), discusses Magendie's role in the development of pharmacology. Olmsted also devotes attention to Claude Bernard's pharmacological work in *Claude Bernard: Physiologist* (New York: Harper and Brothers, 1939) and, coauthored with E. Harris Olmsted, *Claude Bernard and the Experimental Method in Medicine* (New York: Henry Schuman, 1952).

On the emergence of pharmacology as an independent discipline in the German-speaking world, see Gustav Kuschinsky, "The Influence of Dorpat on the Emergence of Pharmacology as a Distinct Discipline," *J. Hist. Med.* 23 (1968): 258–71; E. R. Haberman, "Rudolf Buchheim and the Beginnings of Pharmacology as a Science," *Ann. Rev. Pharmacol.* 14 (1974): 1–8; Marianne Bruppacher-Cellier, *Rudolf Buchheim (1820–1879) und die Entwicklung einer experimentellen Pharmakologie* (Zuruck: Julius Druck, 1971); Jan Koch-Weser and Paul J. Schechter, "Schmiedeberg in Strassburg, 1872–1918: The Making of Modern Pharmacology," *Life Sci.* 22 (1978): 1361–72.

John J. Abel

Abel is the central figure in this book, and hence deserves a special category in this essay. The richest source of information on Abel is the John Jacob Abel Papers at the Alan Mason Chesney Medical Archives of the Johns Hopkins Medical Institutions in Baltimore, Maryland. In fact, this collection is the single most valuable source for the book as a whole, as is amply documented in the chapter notes. The collection consists of about 90 linear feet of correspondence, notebooks, photographs, and other materials, housed in 127 manuscript boxes. There are forty-seven boxes of correspondence, ranging from his years as a college student to the end of his life. The early correspondence between Abel and his fiancée and later wife is a valuable resource for both the biographical information that it provides on Abel and the light that it sheds on the education of a physician-scientist in the late nineteenth century. Abel's professional correspondence documents not only his career, but also many aspects of the development of pharmacology in the United States.

There is no book-length biography of Abel, but a number of useful biographical articles about him have been published. The most substantial obituaries (both with bibliographies of Abel's publications) are William deBerniere MacNider, "Biographical Memoir of John Jacob Abel, 1857–1938," *Biog. Mem. Natl. Acad. Sci.* 24 (1947): 231–57 and Carl Voegtlin, "John Jacob Abel, 1857–1938," *J. Pharmacol. Exp. Ther.* 67 (1939): 373–406. *John Jacob Abel, M.D., Investigator, Teacher, Prophet, 1857–1938: A Collection of Papers by and about the Father of American Pharmacology* (Baltimore: Williams and Wilkins, 1957) includes articles on Abel by E. K. Marshall, Jr., and Paul D. Lamson, as well as reproductions of four of Abel's own papers. A special issue of the *Bulletin of the Johns Hopkins Hospital* (vol. 101, no. 6, December 1957) contains recollections of Abel from various periods in his life by seven of his colleagues. See also Charles E. Rosenberg, "John Jacob Abel," *Dictionary of Scientific Biography* (New York: Charles Scribner's Sons, 1970), 1: 9–12.

On Abel's brief tenure on the Michigan faculty, see Henry H. Swain, E. M. K. Geiling, and Alexander Heingartner, "John Jacob Abel at Michigan: The Introduction of Pharmacology into the Medical Curriculum," *Univ. Michigan Med. Bull.* 29 (1963): 1–14. Abel's career at Johns Hopkins is discussed in John Parascandola, "John J. Abel and the Development of Pharmacology at the Johns Hopkins University," *Bull. Hist. Med.* 56 (1982): 512–27 (the information in this article has been incorporated into the present book).

For information on two of Abel's major research contributions, see Jane H. Murnaghan and Paul Talalay, "John J. Abel and the Crystallization of Insulin," *Perspect. Biol. Med.* 10 (1967): 334–80 and Horace W. Davenport, "Epinephrin(e)," *Physiologist* 25 (1982): 76–82.

Academic Pharmacology in the United States

The most useful general work on the teaching of pharmacology in American medical schools is David Cowen, "Materia Medica and Pharmacology," in Ronald L. Numbers, ed., *The Education of American Physicians: Historical Essays* (Berkeley: University of California Press, 1980). The 192 footnotes in Cowen's essay are a valuable source of references on the subject. On pharmacy schools, see John Parascandola and John Swann, "Development of Pharmacology in American Schools of Pharmacy," *Pharm. Hist.* 25 (1983): 95–115 (which provides more detail on the subject than is included in the discussion in this book). On the earlier teaching of materia medica, see J. Hampton Hoch, "A Survey of the Development of Materia Medica in American Schools and Colleges of Pharmacy," *Am. J. Pharm. Educ.* 12 (1948): 148–61. Other professional schools (such as nursing, dentistry, and veterinary medicine) were not significant centers for teaching and research in pharmacology in the period under study in this book and will not be covered in this bibliography, but it should be noted that almost nothing has been written on the history of pharmacology in these institutions.

Several reports or surveys have dealt with the status of pharmacology in medical or pharmacy schools at different times. Perhaps the earliest detailed study was *Report of the Subcommittee on Pharmacology, Toxicology and Therapeutics*, Section 4 of the *Report of the Committee of One Hundred on a Standard Medical Curriculum for Medical Colleges*, Committee on Medical Education Publication No. 46 (Chicago: American Medical Association, 1909). In 1938 the American Society for Pharmacology and Experimental Therapeutics issued a report on "The Role of Pharmacology in the Medical Curriculum," which was published in K. K. Chen, ed., *The American Society for Pharmacology and Experimental Therapeutics, Incorporated: The First Sixty Years, 1908–1969* (Bethesda, Md.: American Society for Pharmacology and Experimental Therapeutics, 1969), pp. 111–19. For a report on pharmacology in medical schools in the 1950s, see Julius Comroe, Jr., ed., *The Teaching of Physiology, Biochemistry, Pharmacology: Report of the First Teaching Institute, Association of American Medical Colleges, Atlantic City, October 19–23, 1953*, published as part 2 of vol. 29, no. 7 (July 1954) of the *Journal of Medical Education*. With respect to pharmaceutical education, see A. Richard Bliss, "Pharmacodynamics in the Schools and Colleges of Pharmacy," *J. Am. Pharm. Assoc.* 9 (1920): 378–87 and James Dille, "A Study of the Teaching of Pharmacology in Colleges of Pharmacy," *Am. J. Pharm. Educ.* 2 (1938): 8–31.

Two useful published surveys of individual pharmacology programs in schools of medicine and pharmacy in the 1970s, which also include some historical information, are Elliott Vesell, ed., *Survey of Pharmacology in Medical Schools of North America* (Nutley, N.J.: Association for Medical School Pharmacology and American Society for Pharmacology and Experimental Therapeutics, 1974) and Tom S. Miya and R. Craig Schnell, eds., *Survey of Pharmacology and Toxicology Departments. II: Schools of Pharmacy in North America* (n.p., 1975).

Two early articles on the teaching of pharmacology in medical schools by leaders in the field are John J. Abel, "On the Teaching of Pharmacology, Materia Medica and Therapeutics in Our Medical Schools," *Philadelphia Med. J.* 6 (1900): 384–90 (reprinted in *John Jacob Abel, M.D., Investigator, Teacher, Prophet*, pp. 57–72) and Torald Sollmann, "The Teaching of Pharmacology and Therapeutics from the Experimental Standpoint," *J.A.M.A.* 39 (1902): 539–46. An important article by a pioneer in the introduction of pharmacology into the pharmacy curriculum is Rufus A. Lyman, "Experimental Pharmacology: An Essential in the Pharmacy Curriculum," *Amer. J. Pharm.* 82 (1910): 510–16.

Various reports on medical and pharmaceutical education also provide some information on the teaching of pharmacology. Of particular interest to the historian are the two influential reports on medical education by Abraham Flexner, *Medical Education in the United States and Canada: A Report to the Carnegie Foundation for the Advancement of Teaching* (New York: Carnegie Foundation for the Advancement of Teaching, 1910), especially pp. 63–65, and *Medical Education: A Comparative Study* (New York: Macmillan Company, 1925), especially pp. 157–58. Among the most useful reports on pharmacy education are W. W. Charters, A. B. Lemon, and Leon M. Monell, *Basic Material for a Pharmaceutical Curriculum* (New York: McGraw Hill, 1927), especially pp. 156–67; Edward C. Eliot, *The General Report of the Pharmaceutical Survey, 1946–49* (Washington, D.C.: American Council on Education, 1950), especially pp. 98–118; Lloyd E. Blauch and George L. Webster, *The Pharmaceutical Curriculum: A Report Prepared for the Committee on Curriculum, American Association of Colleges of Pharmacy* (Washington, D.C.: American Council on Education, 1952), especially pp. 122–34.

General histories of medical and pharmaceutical education in the United States provide very little information on the teaching of pharmacology (with the exception of the previously cited essay by David Cowen in Numbers, ed., *Education of American Physicians*). These works are essential sources, however, for placing pharmacology within the broader context of the education of American physicians and pharmacists. The best studies of American medical education are Kenneth M. Ludmerer, *Learning to Heal: The Development of American Medical Education* (New York: Basic Books, 1985), and William G. Rothstein, *American Medical Schools and the Practice of Medicine: A History* (New York: Oxford University Press, 1987). On pharmaceutical education, see Glenn Sonnedecker, "American Pharmaceutical Education before 1900" (Ph.D. diss., University of Wisconsin–Madison, 1952), and Robert Mrtek, "Pharmaceutical Education in these United States: An Interpretive Essay of the Twentieth Century," *Am. J. Pharm. Educ.* 40 (1976): 339–65 (reprinted as a separate booklet by the American Association of Colleges of Pharmacy, Bethesda, Md., 1976).

Histories of individual schools of medicine and pharmacy provide some information about the development of pharmacology at these institutions, although in most cases (especially in the pharmacy school histories) the discussions are very brief and general. No attempt will be made here to list all of these histories, but those having substantial information on pharmacology include: Henry K. Beecher and Mark D. Altschule, *Medicine at Harvard: The First Three Hundred Years* (Hanover, N.H.: University Press of New England, 1977), pp. 154–55, 255–64; A. McGhee Harvey, Gert H. Brieger, Susan L. Abrams, and Victor A. McKusick, *A Model of Its Kind. Volume I. A Centennial History of Medicine at Johns Hopkins* (Baltimore: Johns Hopkins Press, 1989), pp. 29–30, 255–58, 309–15; Horace W. Davenport, *Fifty Years*

of Medicine at the University of Michigan, 1891–1941 (Ann Arbor: University
of Michigan Medical School, 1986), pp. 111–34; J. Arthur Myers, *Masters
of Medicine: An Historical Sketch of the College of Medical Sciences University
of Minnesota 1886–1966* (St. Louis: Warren H. Green, 1968), pp. 551–70;
W. Reece Berryhill, William B. Blythe, and Isaac Manning, *Medical Education at Chapel Hill: The First Hundred Years* (Chapel Hill: University of
North Carolina School of Medicine, 1979), pp. 24, 43–50, 54, 132–33; *The
University of Texas Medical Branch at Galveston: A Seventy-five Year History
by the Faculty and Staff* (Austin: University of Texas Press, 1967), pp. 32–
36, 118–19, 257–58, 317; Paul F. Clark, *The University of Wisconsin Medical
School: A Chronicle 1848–1948* (Madison: University of Wisconsin Press,
1967), pp. 95–104.

Two pharmacology programs have been the subject of book-length stud-
ies, namely, B. V. Rama-Sastry, *Pharmacology at Vanderbilt: A Century of
History and Progress, 1875–1975* (Nashville: Vanderbilt University, 1978),
and Chalmers L. Gemmill and Mary Jeanne Jones, *Pharmacology at the
University of Virginia School of Medicine* (Charlottesville: Department of
Pharmacology, University of Virginia, 1966). A booklet on the Michigan program is Henry H. Swain, *One Hundred Years of Pharmacology 1891–1991
Centennial The University of Michigan* (Ann Arbor: University of Michigan,
1991). The notes to chapter 4 provide citations to many other published
sources of information on academic pharmacology programs, but additional
articles include: Earl Dearborn, "The Development of Pharmacology at Boston University School of Medicine," *Boston Med. Q.* 6 (1955): 33–37; P. K.
Knoefel, "History of the Department of Physiology and Pharmacology," *Ken-
tucky Med. J.* 35 (1937): 141–44; Carl A. Dragstedt, "The Department of
Pharmacology: Northwestern Medical School," *Q. Bull. Northwestern Med.
Sch.* 26 (1952): 61–64.

The medical school pharmacology departments at Chicago, Illinois, Vanderbilt, Western Reserve, and Yale in the 1920s and early 1930s were described in articles in *Methods and Problems of Medical Education*, a series
of reports issued by the Rockefeller Foundation. These reports were reprinted
in Alan Gregg, ed., *Reprints from "Methods in Medical Education: Physiology, Pharmacology, and Physiological Chemistry* (New York: Rockefeller
Foundation, 1932).

The catalogues of medical and pharmacy schools are rich sources of information about the development of pharmacology at these institutions. The
National Library of Medicine has a large collection of American medical school
catalogues of the nineteenth and twentieth centuries. The F. B. Power Phar-
maeutical Library at the University of Wisconsin–Madison has a similar excellent collection of catalogues from pharmacy schools.

Book-length biographies do not exist for any of the early leaders in American academic pharmacology. The notes to chapter 4, however, provide ci-

tations to some of the most substantive biographical articles on these individuals.

The personal papers of academic pharmacologists and related manuscript materials are major primary sources for historians of pharmacology. The collections discussed here are mainly those that have proved most useful for this study. None of the other collections of personal papers or departmental records that I have consulted, however, match the richness and significance of the John J. Abel Papers, which were considered in the previous section.

The Alfred Newton Richards Papers at the University of Pennsylvania Archives in Philadelphia consist of forty-two boxes of his correspondence, lecture and research notes, and so forth, mainly from the 1920s through the 1950s. The University of Pennsylvania Archives also houses the papers of Richards's colleague and successor, Carl F. Schmidt. The Medical School Pharmacology and Toxicology Papers at the University of Wisconsin–Madison consist of about fifty-seven boxes of material from the establishment of the department in 1907 up to the early 1960s. The most useful parts of the collection for historical purposes are those containing correspondence, research notebooks, and so forth of Arthur Loevenhart (four boxes) and Arthur Tatum (eight boxes). The State Historical Society of Wisconsin in Madison also has a collection of five boxes of Arthur L. Tatum Papers. The William deBerniere MacNider Papers in the Southern Historical Collections at the Wilson Library, University of North Carolina at Chapel Hill, consist of sixty-three boxes of mostly correspondence. The material dates mainly from the 1920s and 1930s. The Historical Division of the Cleveland Health Sciences Library has a collection of Torald Sollman Papers which is of interest, but it is disappointingly lacking in materials from the earlier period of Sollman's career. The archival records of the Harvard Medical School in the Francis A. Countway Library in Boston include only one box of Reid Hunt Papers, although there are seventeen boxes of materials of his successor, Otto Krayer. The Michigan Historical Collections in the Bentley Historical Library, University of Michigan, Ann Arbor, contain one box of Charles Wallis Edmunds Papers. Although the Chauncey Leake Papers at the National Library of Medicine, consisting of seventy-nine boxes and three bound volumes, were not especially useful for my project since most of the material dates from the post-1940 portion of Leake's career, this collection could be a valuable source for the history of pharmacology beginning in the mid-twentieth century.

University archives also contain other collections that can yield significant information about the development of pharmacology at that institution. For example, the papers of some university presidents (such as those of Daniel Coit Gilman at Johns Hopkins and James Angell at Michigan) were of value in my research. The minutes of groups such as medical school faculties or university boards of trustees also helped me to document key events in some cases.

Another significant manuscript source on the history of academic pharmacology is a collection at the Rockefeller Foundation Archives, RG2 200 American Medical Schools—Pharmacology. This collection consists of a series of letters giving budgets, staffs, and other information about some twenty-five medical school pharmacology programs. The letters were sent to Alan Gregg of the Rockefeller Foundation in response to his 1939 request for this information as part of an effort to call attention to what Gregg felt was inadequate support of pharmacology in most American medical schools. The Rockefeller Foundation Archives also contain information on pharmacology grants awarded to various academic researchers.

Pharmacology in the Federal Government

On the early history of this subject, see John Parascandola, "The Beginnings of Pharmacology in the Federal Government," *Pharm. Hist.* 30 (1988): 179–87 (which has largely been incorporated into chapter 5 of this book). On the Division of Pharmacology of the Hygienic Laboratory (later the National Institutes of Health), see Ralph Chester Williams, *The United States Public Health Service: 1798–1950* (Washington, D.C.: Commissioned Officers Association of the United States Public Health Service, 1951), especially p. 24, and Victoria A. Harden, *Inventing the NIH: Federal Biomedical Research Policy, 1887–1937* (Baltimore: Johns Hopkins University Press, 1986), especially pp. 19–25. The Public Health Service Records (Record Group 90) in the National Archives in Washington, D.C. contain some correspondence of the division, especially in General File (1897–1923), boxes 75 (660) and 98 (1078).

T. Swann Harding's *Two Blades of Grass: A History of Scientific Development in the U.S. Department of Agriculture* (Norman, Okla.: University of Oklahoma Press, 1947) contains little specific information on pharmacology in the department, but see pp. 317–18. The annual reports of the Bureau of Chemistry, the Bureau of Animal Industry, and the Bureau of Plant Industry can be useful sources of information. Pharmacology was especially important in the Bureau of Chemistry because of the bureau's role in the regulation of foods and drugs. The annual reports of the bureau up to 1927, when the responsibility for enforcement of the food and drug law was transferred to the newly-created Food and Drug Administration, are collected together in *Federal Food, Drug and Cosmetic Law: Administrative Reports, 1907–1949* (Chicago: Commerce Clearing House, 1951). The Records of the Bureau of Chemistry (Record Group 97), the Bureau of Animal Industry (Record Group 17) and the Bureau of Plant Industry (Record Group 54) at the National Archives also contain some relevant materials.

A. J. Lehman, "Some Functions of the Division of Pharmacology of the Food and Drug Administration," *Food Drug Cos. Law J.* 7 (1953): 405–16, describes the FDA's pharmacological unit as it functioned in the early 1950s. The annual reports of the FDA, which provide significant information on its pharmacological activities, have been collected together in the previously cited *Administrative Reports, 1907–1949* and in *Food and Drug Administration: Annual Reports, 1950–1974* (Washington, D.C.: Department of Health, Education and Welfare, 1976). The Records of the Food and Drug Administration (Record Group 88) are an important resource, but most post-1938 records are still in the possession of the agency (contact the FDA History Office). The transcript and tapes of "Oral History of the U. S. Food and Drug Administration: Pharmacology" (a 1980 interview with four retired FDA pharmacologists) are in the History of Medicine Division of the National Library of Medicine. The role of FDA pharmacologists in the study of the toxicity of food colors is discussed in Sheldon Hochheiser, "Synthetic Food Colors in the United States: A History under Regulation" (Ph.D. diss., University of Wisconsin–Madison, 1982). On the involvement of pharmacologists in the FDA's efforts to control lead arsenate pesticide spray residues on fruit, see James Whorton, *Before Silent Spring: Pesticides and Public Health in Pre-DDT America* (Princeton: Princeton University Press, 1974), pp. 155–60, 223–31.

For information on pharmacology in the Chemical Warfare Service of the United States Army, see Daniel P. Jones, "The Role of Chemists in Research on War Gases in the United States during World War I" (Ph.D. dissertation, University of Wisconsin–Madison, 1969), especially pp. 92–165, and Stephen A. Gross, "The Formation and Function of the Pharmacological and Toxicological Section, Research Division, Chemical Warfare Service, U. S. Army" (unpublished M.A. paper, Department of the History of Science, University of Wisconsin–Madison, 1982). The Records of the Chemical Warfare Service (Record Group 175) are in the National Archives. The Loevenhart Papers at the University of Wisconsin (cited above) contain some information on the pharmacological and toxicological work of the Chemical Warfare Service in World War I.

Pharmacology in the American Pharmaceutical Industry

Two recent books that discuss the introduction of science into the American pharmaceutical industry and the beginnings of the industry's collaboration with academic scientists are Jonathan Liebenau, *Medical Science and Medical Industry: The Formation of the American Pharmaceutical Industry* (Baltimore: Johns Hopkins University Press, 1987), and John P. Swann, *Academic Scientists and the Pharmaceutical Industry: Cooperative Research in Twentieth-Century America* (Baltimore: Johns Hopkins University Press, 1988). Pharmacology and pharmacologists receive attention in both books, especially in Swann's monograph.

For an overview of the early development of research, including some discussion of pharmacological research, see Malcolm Keith Weikel and Glenn Sonnedecker, "Emergence of Research as a Function of the American Pharmaceutical Industry" (unpublished manuscript, American Institute of the History of Pharmacy, Madison, 1963). (This is a revised version of Malcolm Keith Weikel, "Research as a Function of American Pharmaceutical Industry: The American Formative Period," M.S. diss., University of Wisconsin–Madison, 1962). Peter Stechl, "Biological Standardization of Drugs before 1928" (Ph.D. diss., University of Wisconsin–Madison, 1969), also provides information on early pharmacological research in the American pharmaceutical industry. On the development of research, including pharmacological research, between the two World Wars, see John Parascandola. "Industrial Research Comes of Age: The American Pharmaceutical Industry, 1920–1940," *Pharm. Hist.* 27 (1985): 12–21.

Histories of individual companies tend to be celebratory rather than critical in approach, and in general they are poorly documented. Nevertheless, these works can provide some information on pharmacological research in drug firms, although discussions of the subject are usually relatively brief. Among the more substantial company histories are: Herman Kogan, *The Long White Line* (New York: Random House, 1963), especially pp. 119–30, 215–32 (on Abbott Laboratories); E. J. Kahn, *All in a Century: The First Hundred Years of Eli Lilly and Company* (Indianapolis: Eli Lilly, 1975), especially pp. 109–25; Jeffrey L. Sturchio, ed., *Values and Visions: A Merck Century* (Rahway, N.J.: Merck and Co., 1991); Samuel Mines, *Pfizer: An Informal History* (New York: Pfizer, 1978); John Francis Marion, *The Fine Old House* (Philadelphia: SmithKline Corporation, 1980); Leonard Engel, *Medicine Makers of Kalamazoo* (New York: McGraw-Hill, 1961), especially pp. 49–79, 92–214 (on Upjohn Company). See also James H. Madison, *Eli Lilly: A Life, 1885–1977* (Indianapolis: Indiana Historical Society, 1989).

House organs, company reports, and other industry publications sometimes yield useful information on pharmacology in industry. An extensive historical collection of such materials may be found in the Kremers Reference Files, F. B. Power Pharmaceutical Library, University of Wisconsin–Madison. The archives of the major pharmaceutical firms are of interest to the historian, although these are not always well organized or readily accessible to the public, even when significant historical materials have been preserved. It is necessary to write a company in advance to determine what materials may be available on a given subject and what restrictions have been placed on their use. The most useful industrial archives for my purposes in this study were those of Eli Lilly and Company in Indianapolis and Merck and Company in Rahway, N.J.

The personal papers of academic pharmacologists who had significant ties with industry can be a useful source of information on pharmacology in the commercial sector. The previously mentioned A. N. Richards Papers, for example, are a rich source on the history of pharmacological research at Merck and Company and Richards's involvement with it from the 1930s through the 1950s. The Tatum and Loevenhart Papers (cited above) are also of value with respect to documenting their relationships with pharmaceutical companies.

For a discussion of the national pharmacological society's policy against admitting industrial scientists as members, see John Parascandola, "The 'Preposterous Provision': The American Society for Pharmacology and Experimental Therapeutics' Ban on Industrial Pharmacologists, 1908–1941," in Jonathan Liebenau, Gregory J. Higby, and Elaine C. Stroud, *Pill Peddlers: Essays on the History of the Pharmaceutical Industry* (Madison: American Institute of the History of Pharmacy, 1990), pp. 29–47 (much of which has been incorporated into this book).

A National Society and Journal

On the history of the major national society of professional pharmacologists, see K. K. Chen, ed., *The American Society for Pharmacology and Experimental Therapeutics, Incorporated: The First Sixty Years, 1908–1969* (Bethesda, Md.: American Society for Pharmacology and Experimental Therapeutics, 1969). This volume is more of a chronicle than a history of the society, but it is an invaluable source of information on the meetings, membership, officers, publications, and so forth of the organization. Since 1959, many of the society's activities have been recorded in *The Pharmacologist*, a quarterly (originally semiannual) publication.

The small archives of the American Society for Pharmacology and Experimental Therapeutics in Bethesda, Maryland, is a valuable resource for the study of the society's history. Among the most interesting materials historically are one volume of correspondence dealing with the origins of the society and nine volumes of "Minutes and Records" of the society covering the period from 1908 to 1950. The previously mentioned Abel Papers contain a significant amount of material on the founding and early history of the society.

The first American journal of pharmacology was the *Journal of Pharmacology and Experimental Therapeutics*, founded in 1909 by Abel and still being published today by the American Society for Pharmacology and Experimental Therapeutics. For a brief history of the journal, see Maurice Seevers, "Publications," in Chen, ed., *The American Society*, pp. 123–31. The Abel Papers provide a good deal of information about the journal during the period of Abel's editorship (through 1932). The society's archives also are a useful source of information on this journal.

Useful guides to the periodical literature of pharmacology and toxicology are as follows: George M. Hocking, *Serials Pertaining to Pharmacognosy and*

Pharmacology (New York: S. B. Pernick and Company, 1944); Charles W. Shilling and Mildred Benton, *Pharmacology, Toxicology and Cosmetic Serials: Their Identification and an Analysis of Their Characteristics* (Washington, D.C.: Biological Sciences Communication Project, George Washington University, 1965); Henry Kissman, "Information Retrieval in Toxicology," *Annu. Rev. Pharmacol. Toxicol.* 20 (1980): 285–305; and Phillip Wexler, *Information Resources in Toxicology*, 2d ed. (New York: Elsevier, 1988).

INDEX

Page numbers in italics denote illustrations.

Designed by David denBoer
Composed by the EPS Group, Inc. in Caledonia
Printed by the Princeton University Press
on 50-lb. Glatfelter Vellum Offset
and bound in Holliston Roxite